48 Hours to Kickstart Healthy Weight Loss

Suzi Grant worked as a broadcast journalist for over twenty years before training as a nutritional therapist. She is now a well-known health expert and nutritionist, and a member of the Guild of Health Writers and of the British Association of Nutritional Therapists. She writes regularly for health magazines and appears in the national press and on TV and radio, as well as running workshops around the country and practices in West London and Brighton.

Her first book, *48 Hours to a Healthier Life*, was published by Penguin in 2003. You can find more information about Suzi Grant on her website: www.benatural.co.uk

48 Hours to Kickstart Healthy Weight Loss

Suzi Grant

MICHAEL JOSEPH
an imprint of
PENGUIN BOOKS

Disclaimer: The contents of this book have been carefully researched, but are not intended as a substitute for taking proper medical advice. If you have any acute or chronic disease or are taking medication, you should always consult a qualified doctor or health practitioner. The author and the publisher accept no liability for damage of any nature resulting directly or indirectly from the application or use of information in this book.

MICHAEL JOSEPH

Published by the Penguin Group
Penguin Books Ltd, 80 Strand, London WC2R 0RL, England
Penguin Group (USA) Inc., 375 Hudson Street, New York, New York 10014, USA
Penguin Books Australia Ltd, 250 Camberwell Road, Camberwell, Victoria 3124, Australia
Penguin Books Canada Ltd, 10 Alcorn Avenue, Toronto, Ontario, Canada M4V 3B2
Penguin Books India (P) Ltd, 11 Community Centre, Panchsheel Park, New Delhi – 110 017, India
Penguin Group (NZ), Cnr Airborne and Rosedale Roads, Albany, Auckland 1310, New Zealand
Penguin Books (South Africa) (Pty) Ltd, 24 Sturdee Avenue, Rosebank 2196, South Africa

Penguin Books Ltd, Registered Offices: 80 Strand, London WC2R 0RL, England

www.penguin.com

First published 2004
1

Set in 11.75/14.75 pt Minion
Typeset by Rowland Phototypesetting Ltd, Bury St Edmunds, Suffolk
Printed in Great Britain by Clays Ltd, St Ives plc

A CIP catalogue record for this book is available from the British Library

ISBN 0-718-14748-0

Contents

Warning

If you are on any form of medication, chronically ill, pregnant, severely underweight or overweight, or at all concerned about your health, please seek professional advice before embarking on any of the weight-loss plans, including the 48-Hour Kickstart Detox Weekend.

Foreword

The idea for this book grew, organically, whilst I was writing my first book: *48 Hours to a Healthier Life*. At that time, my clients were constantly coming to the clinic asking for a quick route to 'healthier' weight loss. Meanwhile, the more I sat on my bottom writing, the more weight I put on, despite following an extremely healthy regime! My clients were getting slimmer and healthier and were delighted with the results while I was getting less and less enamoured with the first signs of middle age – right around my middle.

I was brimming with health but my fat stores were telling another story. I knew, just as anyone picking up this book knows, that losing weight isn't rocket science. It's very, very simple: **eat less and exercise more**. But I wasn't doing any of it because I had the perfect excuse – I *had* to sit at my laptop writing for most of every day.

A year on and that extra half a stone has gone and, more importantly, I've gone down a dress size and toned more than I could ever have imagined possible for someone of my age. And I'm still glued to my laptop! The main difference is that I constantly follow one of the three plans in this book and I've found an exercise that is an absolute JOY to do every single day. I eat less and definitely exercise more and I detox regularly.

I still have great weekends eating out with friends and having a few drinks – and so do my clients. But each of us has found the right plan to follow for the rest of the week so the weight *stays* off.

There is no quick fix when it comes to the battle of the bulge. But the one thing I and my clients have found to be essential for permanent and healthy weight loss is to kick off any regime with a detox: a simple 48-hour plan that helps the body let go of toxicity and water quickly and safely. And so the idea for *48 Hours to Kickstart Healthy Weight Loss* was born.

For anyone with a holiday coming up, a sedentary lifestyle, middle-age spread, postnatal bulges or just a few extra pounds to lose that weren't there this time last year, this book's for you. The 48-Hour Plan will kickstart your body to get rid of bloating and water retention just in time for you to get ready to hit the beach in that bikini.

For those who have more than a few pounds to shift, this book is also for you. After you have completed your 48-Hour Kickstart Detox there are **three** long-term plans to choose from which will not only help you lose weight safely at the recommended 2–3 lb a week, but also healthily. So you can improve your chances of avoiding all the conditions now associated with being overweight such as heart disease, diabetes and some cancers.

My clients have been the guinea pigs and every single one who has followed one of the suggested plans, as well as exercising DAILY, has had remarkable success. And so have I! More importantly, we have all experienced other fabulous benefits, such as increased energy, better moods, and smoother skin and less cellulite, along with permanent weight loss.

I dedicate this book to my wonderful clients who have inspired me as much as I hope I have inspired them. It has been a journey we have made together and one that has been so successful it must be shared with the rest of the world!

Testimonials

I no longer want to kill someone if I'm five minutes late for lunch and my bloaty belly is much more under control . . . !   Harriet

Yes! Yes! Yes! Success at last, I have lost 4–5 lb in weight and have kept it off. Many thanks.   Eve

I wore a suit the other day I had not worn for two years.   Ann

My thrush has gone and I have lost half a stone without even trying. I'm eating loads more than I was when I was trying to lose weight.   Simone

Both Mum and I felt so good on it that we are trying to keep it up (obviously HAD to reintroduce the alcohol and a little salt occasionally).   Clare

Kept up daily yoga practice and started fast walking. My weight went down from 9 st 3 lb to 8 st 3 lb in just two months.   Helen

I tried a load of old 'thinner' clothes on over the weekend and I'm only a couple of pounds away from getting into my favourite snakiest pair of jeans.   Deb

My skin is a million times clearer and I'm sure my cellulite is disappearing. Why didn't I find you years ago!   Mrs Brenner

I managed to shift the weight I wanted and have subsequently managed to keep it off! Thanks.   Nicola

1.

Introduction

We are all obsessed by our weight – especially in the summer when it comes to wearing a bikini or shorts for the first time that year. Some of us are just a few pounds overweight while some of us (nearly half of all Britons) are officially overweight.

A survey conducted by Taylor Nelson Sofres for Adios, the herbal slimming product, showed that 44 per cent of us are unhappy with our weight with nearly a quarter of all British women (24 per cent) constantly on a diet, despite the fact that 78 per cent of us don't believe that 'fad' diets actually work!

It doesn't help that supermodels, TV and movie stars, and singers all look fantastic, whatever faddy diet they're following. But don't forget they have an army of make-up and hair artists, personal trainers, and lifestyle coaches to make them look the very best they can. Their livelihood depends on it. Even they suffer from the 'my tummy looks big in this' syndrome.

You know, as well as I, that yo-yo dieting doesn't work. In fact you just stash on even more weight because your body is fooled into thinking you've been starving, so it makes sure you don't starve again by laying down *more* fat for the next time. The only healthy and effective long-range weight-reduction plan is to find a balanced eating plan FOR YOU as an individual. As well as the right lifestyle that will help you reach and stay at your perfect weight.

What can you do in just 48 hours?

We all know that it is impossible to lose *real* weight in just 48 hours. But if you take just 2 days out and dedicate the time to kickstarting your system with a simple detox you WILL lose INCHES as the detox clears toxins from your bloated tummy. You will feel and look better as a couple of POUNDS of toxicity exit your body. And you will find that your clothes fit better as your body releases PINTS of water that it's been holding on to. Detoxification clears toxins from the body by neutralizing them and transforming them into excess water, and the more water you lose, the more inches you lose. You won't be losing weight; you'll be losing waste!

You can either think of the 48-Hour Plan as a kickstart to successful long-term weight loss – the first programme you are really going to succeed at. Or you can treat it as a one-off detox to help you eliminate water retention and bloating fast to get into that size-12 dress. Or both. The choice is yours. All I ask is that you try it!

The 48-Hour Kickstart Detox is designed for you to take time out for yourself so you can experiment with different exercises, foods and techniques. There is no calorie-counting, you don't need to weigh food or weigh yourself and there are no complicated recipes to follow.

And it's not just about what you put in your mouth. You are also going to be able to experiment with emotional, physical and holistic techniques. A step-by-step guide that has been specifically designed with detoxing and eliminating water retention in mind, all to be carried out in the privacy of your own home for a fraction of the price of a blue chip health spa.

Think of it as your home-from-home 'fat farm' where you take charge of your own 'regime' and decide to do something about those extra pounds once and for all. Hopefully, you will feel so energized and look so much better by the end of the weekend that you will be encouraged to carry on with one of the three suggested plans for losing weight safely and effectively at the recommended 1–2 lb a week. And this time keeping it off for ever.

Have a quick look at this list and decide which of the special events coming up requires a flatter tummy and is worth you taking a weekend off to get your body, mind and spirit into the best possible shape.

Special Events

- Wedding
- Family celebration
- New job
- Hot date
- Weekend away
- Minor operation
- Beach holiday
- Birthday
- Party
- Milestone birthday
- Christening
- Activity holiday
- First sign of summer
- Starting a long-term weight-loss plan

Even if you don't have a major event you need to look svelte for, you might just decide that enough is enough and your body needs a really good spring-clean because of:

- Cellulite
- Dull hair
- Dry skin
- Low energy
- Stressful job
- Constant colds
- Permanent bloating
- Hormonal problems
- Middle-age spread
- Postnatal blues

If you want a long-term weight-loss plan

If, after following the 48-Hour Plan, you want to continue to lose a steady 2 lb a week of *real* weight safely, easily and healthily, you are far more likely to succeed if you have done the Kickstart Detox first.

There are three plans for you to choose from but, as this is YOUR health spa, you can always change your mind and switch to another plan or even try each of them one after another. It's your book, your body, and your choice!

DETOX – you carry on with the detox for a *maximum* of 6 weeks and give your body the best possible chance of a real cleanse.

SLIMMER'S SMOOTHIES – you replace up to two meals a day

with a smoothie power-packed with everything your body needs nutritionally.

HIGH-PROTEIN, LOW-CARB – the emphasis is on HEALTHY protein and low-carbohydrate intake for maximum weight loss and energy.

Different plans will suit different people, depending on your own individual taste, pocket and lifestyle. Answering the questions below will help steer you towards the right eating plan for all sorts of conditions, from hormonal problems to fluctuating blood-sugar levels, as well as losing weight. You may also have a quick look at each of the plans in chapters 14, 15 and 16 to see if one of them jumps out at you as something you can live with. I'm a great believer in intuition and it's often how I work with my clients. I think you will know instinctively which one you can live with in the real world.

The one thing that all 3 plans have in common is that they are safe, healthful and do-able for as long as you like. The word 'diet' comes from the Latin *diaeta* and the Greek *diaita*, meaning 'way of life' or 'regimen'. It shouldn't be something you do for 2–3 months then stop, it should be a 'life plan' with plenty of treats built-in so you never, ever feel deprived. So you won't see the word 'diet' cropping up too often because we know they don't work, don't we?

You don't need to worry about what these plans might do to your long-term health either. You can only get healthier, slimmer and fitter on these plans. And, more importantly, THEY WORK.

You may now like to sit down with a pen and fill in the quizzes to see which of the 3 plans is most likely to benefit you – the more ticks you have, the more suited to that particular plan you are.

A – Carry on with the Detox

I get up every night to urinate
I don't move my bowels every day
I have aches and pains in my muscles and joints

I crave salty foods such as cheese, crisps and olives
I take painkillers for headaches every week
I have cellulite
I live on fast food and takeaways
I drink alcohol every night
I have IBS symptoms
I often suffer from indigestion

B – Slimmer's Smoothies

I have dry hair, scalp and skin
My blood pressure is high
I exercise regularly but can't lose weight
I suffer from hormonal problems
I need more energy
I often get the blues
I often feel tired and lethargic
I suffer from skin problems such as acne and eczema
My nails are very brittle and flaky
I feel under the weather

C – High-protein, Low-carb

I feel very groggy in the morning
I feel irritable if I miss a meal
I have a family history of adult-onset diabetes
I often crave alcohol, cigarettes or coffee
I crave chocolate regularly
I crave starchy foods such as bread, bananas and potatoes
I have no time to prepare special meals
I eat out regularly
I suffer the afternoon slumps
I often eat when I'm not hungry

Results

Mostly As

You really need to carry on with the detox (with some welcome additions) for a *maximum* of 6 weeks. This will give your liver a chance to completely regenerate which, in turn, will help your whole body function better and lose weight more easily. This regime is particularly suited to vegetarians, vegans and readers who like pulses and grains. The plan will also increase your immunity and give you all the benefits you can expect from a detox, as well as weight loss.

Mostly Bs

Your answers point to a body needing far more essential fatty acids than you are providing it with. During this plan you will be replacing two of your daily meals with a nutrient-packed and ridiculously filling smoothie that you make yourself. If you go out to work each day, you can have a smoothie for breakfast, a proper lunch as your main meal and a smoothie for supper. It will certainly suit those of you who prefer shakes or smoothies to sit-down meals and who want to burn fat fast.

Mostly Cs

This is the easiest plan to follow long-term whether you are a manic mum with a family or a busy executive who eats out all the time. Blood-sugar level problems and Candida symptoms should vanish on this plan as it consists of very healthy proteins and low carbohydrates, not *no* carbohydrates. This is a plan you can follow for life, quite safely.

If you have an equal mixture of As, Bs and Cs, wait till you have finished reading the book before deciding. There is absolutely nothing to stop you from trying each of them at different times. All I ask, for maximum results, is that you KICKSTART any plan you choose with the 48-Hour Detox. All will be revealed in the next chapter: Why do I need to detox and how do I prepare?

2.

Why a Kickstart Detox Weekend

If you're in a real hurry to start, you can go straight to the Kickstart Detox Weekend, chapter 13. But if you can spare the time, I would recommend that you read through the following brief chapters on **W-E-I-G-H-T L-O-S-S** so you can discover WHY this detox is going to help kickstart your metabolism, before we get into HOW.

W – Weight: in this chapter you will learn *why* we put on weight, whether we're young, middle-aged or old. There's a test to see if you really are overweight and an explanation on how metabolism works.

E – Eliminate: here we look at why certain foods and drinks encourage our bodies to store fat and why it's so important to do without them for as long as possible in order to promote weight loss.

I – Incorporate: this chapter will give you an idea of the alternative foods and drinks you can have that will actively encourage water- and weight loss quickly.

G – Get Up and Go: You *cannot* lose weight effectively without exercise and here we explore how much exercise, and how often, you need to encourage your body to burn fat and not muscle.

H – Holistic Therapies are very useful to help shift water and kickstart your system to lose weight. This chapter explores which therapies have the best results and why.

T – Toxicity in the cells encourages your body to hang on to fat, however little you eat. Learn how 'life' in general could be affecting your weight.

L – Liver: here you will see why the liver is thought of as the most important organ in the body when it comes to losing weight.

O – Oedema: otherwise known as water retention; this chapter explains why cells hang on to water and what causes it.

S – Synergy: maybe you need a little bit more than exercise and diet. Here we explore other techniques such as visualization and affirmations and their role in fighting the flab.

S – Supplements: why supplements can help your weight-loss plan and support your body during a detox.

Why you need to detox to lose weight

Whether you're going straight into the 48-Hour Detox because you've got a special occasion you need to look your best for, or whether you're doing it to prepare your body for a longer weight-loss plan, it's important to know *why* detoxing will help you.

Excess weight or inches is very often just waste that is stuck in the colon or stored as fat in the tissues: where the body just loves to stash pesticides, food additives and toxins. Too much toxicity and your clever body hangs on to water to keep any toxic material away from your vital organs. Which is why you can appear to have put on 6 lb the morning after a night out boozing, eating and smoking. It isn't real weight, you couldn't possibly put on that much weight in 12 hours. It's just water and toxicity. And you can lose a lot of it in just 48 hours.

Liver overload

Stimulants and toxins throw the body's metabolic balance into upheaval and give the liver so much work to do that it can't keep up with detoxing and filtering all the stuff we throw at it. A healthy, clean liver will metabolize your food much more efficiently and you are more likely to burn fat. The longer you detox the better your liver will work, but you can kickstart it into cleansing in just 48 hours.

Adrenal overload

Salt, sugar, coffee, alcohol, and stress all over-stimulate the adrenals if taken to excess. These two little glands, which sit on top of the kidneys, will then over-stimulate the production of cortisol. This in turn stimulates water retention, inflammation and excess blood glucose. And if it goes on for long, it leads to more water retention and fat storage – especially around the middle!

Cutting down on stress and stimulants will help your blood-sugar levels and get rid of water retention.

Digestion overload

Finally, you need energy to lose weight and the biggest drain on energy is food in the stomach that is hard to digest and assimilate. The more unnatural the food we eat, the harder the digestion has to work and the less energy is left to clear debris out of your body. Result? Your clothes feel tight and your stomach has blown out like a balloon.

In chapter 13, the 48-Hour Kickstart Detox, you will be encouraged to give your digestion as little to do as possible. That way your detoxification process is more likely to lead to successful and permanent weight loss.

How long

Detox programmes can last from one weekend to 6 weeks, depending on your lifestyle. I recommend an initial 48-hour detox before *any* weight-loss programme because anyone can find just 2 days to kickstart the system to become a fat-burning machine! However, if you can cope with doing a detox for longer, 6 weeks is just the very BEST length of time because it takes exactly 6 weeks for your liver to have replaced every single cell with a new healthy cell. The cleaner your liver, the better it will metabolize your food, and the more weight you will lose.

Whether you decide to be brave and extend the 48-Hour Detox for a few weeks or just do the 2 days because you're in a hurry, don't whatever you do rush into it without following the preparation advice at the start of chapter 13. You can't just put a date in your diary and decide on that particular date you are going to give up coffee, chocolate and booze all at once. You will end up feeling terrible and wish you had never started. You need to pre-plan any detox plan and give yourself as much notice as possible. That way your 48 hours will be painless and you will reap the most benefit from it.

You can now go straight to chapter 13, to see what you're in for, or, preferably, have a quick read of the following chapters, starting with weight. Are you really overweight?

3.

W – Weight

Am I overweight?

Just to cheer yourself up, here's a very simple test to see if you really are overweight. And after that I would like you not to look at the scales again but to go for maximum 'inch' loss rather than maximum weight loss.

A healthy weight range is based on a measurement known as the Body Mass Index (BMI), based on your height and weight.

> Work out your height in metres and multiply the figure by itself.
> Measure your weight in kilograms.
> Divide the weight by the height squared (your first figure).

For example: if you are **1.6 m** (5 feet 3 inches) tall and weigh **65 kg** (10 stone) the figures stack up like this:

$1.6 \times 1.6 = 2.56$. The BMI will be 65 divided by 2.56 = **25.39**. Now look at the chart below.

Recommended BMI chart
(based on a woman of average build)

BMI less than 20	Underweight
BMI 20–25	Ideal
BMI 25–30	Overweight
BMI 30–40	Should lose weight
BMI greater than 40	It is essential to lose weight for the sake of your health.

Hopefully, you have been pleasantly surprised and have discovered, as I did, that you are not overweight at all. You just have a little toxicity and water retention to lose!

If you find metric measures a bit of a pain, you can make life much easier for yourself by just going to any of the health websites and searching for BMI. I found a simple version on the BBC website. You will find the address in Resources at the back of the book.

Now let's look at *why* we put on weight.

Weight gain – why do we put on weight?

I would need a whole book to answer this question, there are so many theories around, but here's a list of the most common reasons for piling on the pounds.

- It's My Metabolism
- It's My Age
- Sluggish Liver
- Nutrient Deficiencies
- Underactive Thyroid
- Yeast Infection
- Poor Diet & Digestion
- Food Allergies
- Insulin Resistance – Syndrome X
- It's Emotional
- Happier Than Before
- Unhappier Than Before
- I Have More Fat Cells
- Overeating
- Eating the Children's Leftovers
- Habits
- It's Heredity
- It's Hormonal
- Lack of Exercise
- I Sit at a Desk All Day

Ring any bells? The main reason we put on weight is a combination of two things – eating too many calories and using up too little energy. Not rocket science, as I said before. But *any* of the theories could be linked to a sudden gain around the girth, so let's take a brief look at each of them here. You'll find solutions for all of them from chapter 13 onwards.

● *It's My Metabolism*
● *It's My Age*

It could well be your metabolism or your age, or both!

Research has shown that from your mid-twenties onwards, your metabolism slows down each year. The basal metabolic rate (BMR) – the rate we burn calories at rest – begins to decline from age 25–30 along with the volume of lean muscle tissue. The result is an overall loss in Lean Body Mass (LBM) and a gain in adipose tissue – fatty tissue. However hard you're dieting, unless you're exercising as well, you will automatically lose more than 3 kg of muscle tissue every decade, which results in a 2–5 per cent drop in your metabolic rate every 10 years. That will guarantee a middle-age spread of more than a **stone in fat** by the time you are 45. How unfair is that?

One pound of muscle requires about 35 calories a day just to function, while a pound of fat needs only a couple of calories. So if you want to lose weight, you need to increase your lean muscle mass, big-time. You need to use your muscles to burn fat; there is no other way.

Don't worry, if you follow the suggestions in this book and combine a healthy-eating plan with the right kind of regular exercise you WILL burn fat.

● *Sluggish Liver*
● *Nutrient Deficiencies*

Much like our muscles, the digestive system (and all our other organs) also ages and weakens as we get older. Most people will start having digestive problems between 45 and 55, when the body's ability to produce digestive enzymes reduces **by half**. Middle-age spread is very common amongst people with a sluggish liver and poor digestion.

You will find plenty of tips on how to improve your digestion and strengthen your liver later in this book.

● *Underactive Thyroid*

The thyroid gland regulates body metabolism and if it's underactive you may well be putting on unexplained weight. Although an underactive thyroid is becoming more and more common in the West today, a change in diet, nutrients and lifestyle can usually help long before you need to go to the doctor for help.

At the back of the book, you'll find a simple test you can do for yourself at home to find out if your thyroid is or isn't under-functioning. The odds are it isn't but it's worth doing to put your mind at rest. You'll also be given ideas on how best to support your thyroid.

● *Yeast Infection*
● *Poor Diet & Digestion*
● *Food Allergies*

Many people with almost normal body fat readings have big tummies simply because they're carrying around up to *nine* meals' worth of undigested food at any one time.

All of us have more than a kilo of friendly bacteria living in harmony with us each and every day. They're provided with a home and regular meals and, in return, they break down the fibre and waste in the colon and help get everything moving out.

But if someone has consumed a diet of **fast food, meat, milk, sugar, antibiotics and booze** all their lives, the bad bacteria can multiply like mad and upset that balance. Food doesn't get broken down and digested properly and it ends up dumped in the colon where it just sits there and rots. Result? Bloating, gas and that enormous pot belly. The unfriendly bacteria have won!

The 48-Hour Kickstart Detox weekend will help your friendly bacteria start winning the battle, while the long-term detox will help them win the war!

● *Insulin Resistance – Syndrome X*

This has become one of the most fashionable reasons for people piling on the weight, and there must be something in it because any of my clients who exclude carbohydrates high on the glycaemic index (more in chapter 16) *always* lose weight.

Starchy carbs cause the body to release large quantities of the hormone insulin. The more your diet is made up of fast-releasing carbohydrates such as pastries, biscuits and even cornflakes, the more the body has to respond by producing insulin and the more your blood-sugar levels fluctuate. If this goes on indefinitely you put on weight because if you don't burn it off the blood glucose, converted to glycogen, gets stored as fat. Over time, the insulin receptors and the pancreas just get exhausted from the constant demands and insulin resistance sets in.

Help is at hand in chapter 16; the high-protein, low-carb eating plan will sort out your insulin levels once and for all.

● *It's Emotional*
● *Happier Than Before*
● *Unhappier Than Before*

Carrying extra weight has long been associated with the emotions: protecting yourself from being hurt, suffering from a lack of love, a lack of forgiveness etc. No one is happy just because they have a flat stomach and no one is unhappy just because they're overweight. But any spiritual development, such as T'ai Chi Ch'uan, yoga or meditation, can certainly help with emotional issues.

In chapter 11, Synergy, you will learn about exercises to help you cultivate your heart and mind for a healthy perspective on size and weight and you will find inspirational affirmations and positive-thinking exercises in chapter 13 – the 48-Hour Kickstart Detox.

● *I Have More Fat Cells*

We each develop a specific number of fat cells in our body. It may well be genetic but it could also be that we've been overfed at times when we *create* more fat cells: before birth, during childhood and as a growing teenager. Especially the latter, when fat cells get bigger and multiply. If we overeat at this time, the body is more likely to lay down fat in the fat cells and 'puppy fat' develops.

At other times in our adult life we increase only the **size** of our cells, not the number. When we take in more than we use, our cells and fat stores get bigger. Especially the 'white' fat found in the fat cells that lie right under the skin. This is where the body puts extra calories that we haven't used.

When we slim the fat cells get smaller. It's as simple as that!

● *Overeating*
● *Eating the Children's Leftovers*
● *Habits*
● *It's Heredity*

According to a study published in the journal *Psychological Science*, in the US hamburger portions have doubled, pasta servings have quadrupled and chocolate chip cookies are 700 per cent bigger than they were 20 years ago!

The bad news is that the American style of super-size portions has come to the UK and, according to Tim Lang, professor of food policy at City University in London, we need to nip it in the bud now. 'The British are eating more and exercising less. This is silly of us. We have to reverse that trend,' says Lang.

Overweight can also be caused by a habit. It could even be a habit that your mother developed in you. Maybe she made you finish everything on your plate – and you still do.

Have a really good think about what sort of habits you've developed that can lead to overeating. Much as smokers need to identify their triggers, you need to find out what is causing you to snack. Try keeping the SNACK ATTACK diary below for a few days to see if you can get to the root of the problem and then create a diversion.

If, for example, you always snack on the children's leftovers, make it a rule that any scraps go straight into the bin, or the dog, and reward yourself by telephoning a friend instead!

Snack attack diary

When _____

Where _____

What _____

Why _____

What am I Doing at the Time _____

Am I Sitting Down or Standing _____

How Much _____

How Hungry am I _____

How Often am I Snacking _____

The last question on this list is worth considering! If you have a bowl of grapes, nuts or other snacks out on a table, you may well take a handful every time you pass without thinking. Put them away, a handful here and there can soon add up!

● *It's Hormonal*

Menopause expert Dr John Stevenson, from Endocrinology and Metabolic Medicine, Faculty of Medicine, Imperial College in London, says it's already hard for women to maintain a healthy weight after the menopause because of hormonal and metabolic changes. 'Older women tend to carry body fat around the waist in an "apple" shape, much as men do,' says Dr Stevenson. Sadly, the older we get, the more we have to do. 'Post-menopausal women have to eat less and/or exercise more just to *maintain* their weight as they get older. But if you want to **lose** weight, you need to eat less *and* increase activity,' adds Dr Stevenson.

It's also a well-known fact that menstruating women can put on extra weight – fluid retention – before their periods because of hormone fluctuations.

● *Lack of Exercise*
● *I Sit at a Desk All Day*

As you read earlier, muscles burn calories ALL the time, even when we're resting or sitting at a desk all day! Therefore, the more muscle you have, the faster your metabolism will be and the more you will lose weight.

Without exercising regularly (at least 4–5 times a week) you will find it more difficult to lose weight. But it needs to be combined with regular *resistance* training to really kick in. Using weights, or even using your own limbs as weights, is known as muscle-resistant exercise, which *really* burns body fat. The scales may well stay the same as you develop more muscle, but you will lose INCHES from all over your body.

There is a quick and easy muscle-resistant sequence for you in chapter 13, as well as other exercise suggestions that you can incorporate into your normal everyday life in chapter 6 – Get Up and Go.

Hopefully, by now, you are as convinced as me that yo-yo dieting doesn't work (80–90 per cent regain the lost weight and sometimes more), fad diets don't work and dieting without exercising rarely works. This isn't going to happen to you if you follow the advice set out in this book. But you need to change your mind-set, as well as your habits, and decide that this is going to be a *lifetime* plan of 80 per cent healthy eating, 20 per cent a little of what you fancy, with 100 per cent effort when it comes to exercise. That way, I promise you, you'll lose weight safely, healthily and permanently.

Even if none of the above apply and you're young with only a few pounds to lose, it's worth considering changing some of your habits now so you don't find an extra stone of weight's crept on 20 years down the road!

In the next chapter we explore why certain foods have to be banished if we're going to beat the bloat.

4.
E – Eliminate

You need *energy* to detox and lose weight, but the number-one drain on energy – apart from exercise – is digesting what I call 'challenging' food. If you eat something seemingly harmless, such as a wholemeal cheese sandwich, your stomach is going to need a lot of energy digesting it. It might be healthy, but it's fattening and very 'challenging'. The stomach is basically saying, 'I don't have time to get rid of this fluid retention because I'm so busy breaking down this sandwich.' And, surprise, surprise, your body goes into a sudden energy slump within an hour and your belly bloats.

Apart from challenging food, you also need to avoid – for just 2 days – anything that's going to burden your main elimination organs: liver, colon and kidneys. Excessive salt, sugar, diuretics, protein, saturated fat and toxins can all encourage fluid retention because your body needs to mobilize huge amounts of water to remove the stimulants. The body then *retains* water to keep the toxic material away from your vital organs – which is why you can look so puffy.

In order to improve the function of these important organs, so you lose toxicity and water fast, there's a pretty strict exclusion list – but it is only 2 days.

There will be some welcome additions if you do decide to continue your detox for 3–6 weeks.

Exclusion List

- Nicotine & Other Toxins
- Coffee & Tea
- Alcohol
- Sugar

- Artificial Sweeteners
- Salt & Processed Food
- Dairy Products
- Wheat – that includes
  Pasta!
- Potatoes
- Animal Protein: Meat, Fish
  & Eggs etc
- Soya & Pulses

Nicotine & other toxins

You will find a full explanation as to why toxins make you fat in chapter 8, Toxicity. Suffice to say that fat cells just 'love' chemicals and stash them away in places like the back of your thighs to protect you. If you want proof just see which of your friends has the worst cellulite. I'd bet my hat that the smokers in the group suffer from worse cellulite than those who've never smoked do.

Coffee & tea

These are the stimulants we turn to when we need an extra surge of energy and the ones we most crave first thing in the morning to get us going. Coffee, tea and cigarettes stimulate the central nervous system, which is why we feel, temporarily, more lively and alert when we've had our fix.

But, in excess, they have the same effect on your body as sugar, raising your blood-glucose level, increasing your insulin production, producing more glucose and a roller coaster of blood-sugar highs and lows. Regular use of stimulants, far from keeping your weight off, actually programmes you to put on weight in the long run.

Alternatives

Green Tea – a study from the University of Geneva found that green tea could boost your metabolic rate by 4 per cent. It contains a tiny amount of caffeine so is good for those of us who are missing our daily fix.

Dandelion Tea – helps to drain liver and gall bladder so great for a detox.

Nettle Tea – stimulates the kidneys to release more water, naturally.

Herbal Teas – are full of toxin-fighting antioxidants.

Detox Teas – there are many containing detox helpers such as: liquorice, ginger, dandelion, fennel seed and parsley.

Miso Instant Soup – can be bought in sachets and usually contains sea vegetables so is an easy-to-prepare, detoxing hot drink.

Alcohol

It's very simple! Lovely as your favourite cocktail is, alcohol is a diuretic, so the more you drink, the more you pee. The kidneys try to prevent dehydration and compensate by *retaining water* in the body to balance your fluids. Result the next morning? A raging headache and bloating. That's why drinking plenty of water's so important when you're out on the town.

Alcohol is also the most rapidly absorbed sugar you can have and produces excess blood glucose if you drink too much of it. If you're not burning it off, the blood glucose is quickly turned to glycogen and stashed as fat.

Alcohol also stimulates the liver, so we need to give this precious organ a good rest during the detox to give it a chance to concentrate on getting rid of garbage – and some weight.

And for anyone who suspects a yeast overgrowth, as in Candida albicans, drinks such as beer, wine and champagne are especially good at feeding fungal overgrowth because they're fermented.

Need any convincing as to why alcohol needs to be avoided for the 48-Hour Kickstart Detox?

Sugar & artificial sweeteners

Our main source of energy comes from our blood sugar in the form of glucose. Glucose is converted to glycogen, an essential fuel, but we can only store a limited amount in our 'fuel tanks' and if we don't use it we end up storing it as fat.

Refined sugar, in the form of chocolate, sweets or biscuits, encourages our blood-sugar levels to peak too fast and, unless you're an athlete, the glucose produced has nowhere to go and just gets transported to the cells to be laid down as fat.

Honey, syrup, dextrose, sucrose and **fructose** are all forms of sugar and are also turned into glucose quicker than any other foods. So they too can cause the body to store excess fat.

Low-calorie drinks, artificially sweetened, aren't much better. Most health professionals, including me, believe that low-cal drinks may actually encourage weight gain because your taste buds taste 'sugar' and automatically crave even more sugar – in the form of snacks or carbs. More glucose is produced and, again, if it's not used up it just gets stored as fat.

It can't be just a coincidence that the countries buying the most low-calorie drinks have the highest rates of obesity in the world. Obesity has tripled in the UK in the last fifteen years, yet we are eating *fewer* calories and *less* fat and consuming more diet drinks than ever before.

Alternatives

If you really can't live without a little sweetener, try these: Valdivia sugar, brown rice sugar, date sugar.

Salt

Salt, or sodium, is essential for electrolyte balance and without it we would certainly die. But, in excess, salt can severely upset the body's water balance (and cause high blood pressure). Your kidneys filter sodium out of your blood and return the exact amount needed by your body for its electrolyte balance.

But every time your kidneys excrete extra water to deal with an excess of sodium in the blood, *water is retained*. The body is holding on to extra amounts of water to dilute the sodium. The cells become waterlogged and water retention and bloating set in – big-time!

The recommended daily allowance needed for a perfect electrolyte balance is, according to the UK's Food Commission, an average 6 grams per person – just a **small teaspoon**. But most of us consume at least **double** that amount. It's hidden in the most innocent of foods, such as breakfast cereal, ready-made meals and low-fat food.

Alternative

Nature et Progrès Seasalt is harvested by hand with no added chemicals and none of its 80 minerals and electrolytes removed. It is low in organic sodium and has the right ratios of magnesium, potassium, and calcium for an alkaline balance. As it's unrefined, it is grey in colour, and slightly damp. Ask your local health store to get it for you if they don't stock it.

Recommended by Dr Shamim Daya, who specializes in nutritional medicine, this salt is the one exception to the rule because, as she says, 'It is as nature intended and includes essential minerals such as potassium, which will help balance the thyroid and thus your metabolism.'

Dairy products

Although high in calcium, dairy products are also high in saturated fat. They don't really play a part in a healthy weight-loss plan. Not only that, but dairy intolerance is now one of the main food intolerances in the UK. Cow's milk, in particular, can cause excessive mucus and bacteria in the intestines (as well as in the sinuses) which will account for a few extra pounds in weight.

We are the only mammals that drink another mammal's milk

when fully grown and most nutritionists would agree that cow's milk is really meant for calves.

Milk and cheese, in particular, are also very hard to digest – especially cooked cheese – because the pasteurization process prevents the digestive enzymes from doing their work.

And finally, IF the cow has been fed hormones, or antibiotics, they will be passed on to you.

Don't worry, you won't be going short of calcium. There are plenty of calcium-rich alternatives in chapter 13 as well as a couple of dairy surprises that I consider essential for a successful detox.

Alternative calcium-rich foods

Kale, nuts and seeds, especially almonds, parsley, sea vegetables, nettles and all dark green, leafy vegetables.

Dairy products

- Milk
- Margarine
- Cheese
- Evaporated or Condensed Milk
- Ice Cream
- Chocolate

Bread, pasta & potatoes

Wheat is also very hard for many people to digest and is believed to account for 2 per cent of the UK population's allergies. When it comes to wheat *intolerance*, that figure is much higher. According to Allergy UK, a medical charity that helps allergy-sufferers, it could be as many as a quarter of us. Digestive problems such as IBS and bloating are often due to the two insoluble proteins found in wheat – gliadins and glutenins, which produce gluten when the flour is kneaded with water. Any food intolerance can manifest as bloating and water retention.

Even if you don't have a wheat intolerance, most processed bread and pasta tend to contain sugar, salt or additives. Just see how long a cheap sliced loaf lasts compared to a freshly baked baguette. You don't need any of those extra 'toxins' clogging up your fat cells.

Finally, and most importantly for any weight-loss plan, eating too many sandwiches, pasta dishes and other starchy carbs, such as potatoes, causes bloating because starch needs *three times as much water* to convert the starch to glycogen. No wonder your waistline expands and your energy levels slump within an hour of eating.

Think how flour mixed with water turns into a spongy, chewing-gum-like material, which literally sticks to anything. This is what is going on in your gut, so a very good reason to do without it for at least 48 hours.

For rapid fluid elimination, we will be avoiding all starchy carbohydrates during the Weekend Detox.

Animal protein

Although protein is absolutely essential for a healthy body and successful weight loss, animal protein needs to be eliminated during any detox plan because it is, again, hard work for the digestion, needing more energy to be broken down and assimilated. Energy that's needed to detoxify the body.

If protein is not broken down properly, the digestion can become sluggish and toxic and it can take *days* to get a thick, juicy steak out of the body. Fruit and veg are eliminated in a matter of *hours*.

Meat, in particular, is very acid-forming, which will encourage the growth of unfriendly bacteria, adding to your toxic load. Red meat and other meats are also high in arachidonic acid, which encourages inflammation and fluid retention.

Because your digestion needs a weekend off to get its house in order, all animal protein (with one exception) is off the menu – just for 2 days. You will get all the protein you need from nuts and seeds and other alternatives. Protein, animal and non-animal, will be reintroduced in all 3 plans as soon as you've finished your Kickstart Detox.

Soya & pulses

You may be surprised to see these two non-animal proteins on the hit list (apart from a very small amount of soya milk and miso). The reason I've added them is that they may be healthy and a great alternative for vegetarians and vegans, but they can also be mucus-forming and acidic if eaten excessively. Pulses are also very well-known for their bloating ability! So, as it's only 2 days, anything that requires your digestion to work hard is off the menu.

5.

I – Incorporate these Foods

Eat your fruit and veg

These fruit and veg have been specifically chosen because each and every one of them contains an enzyme, compound, vitamin or mineral that will positively encourage your body to excrete sodium and water, help your liver detox, and strengthen your capillaries to *prevent* fluid retention.

Apart from providing all the vitamins and minerals you need, many of these foods are natural diuretics, high in magnesium and potassium, which will help get excess water, sodium and toxicity out of the cells. These are your SUPER FOODS that are really going to boost your energy levels, cleanse your liver and colon and help you banish bloating once and for all.

I could give you a breakdown of what each food contains but, if you're anything like me, your eyes will glaze over after the third reference to folic acid or bioflavonoids! So I've made it simple with a short description of what each food actually *does* for you during a detox.

Meanwhile, here's a reminder of why eating your veg is going to help you lose weight in just 48 hours.

Vegetable facts

- Four times as much potassium and magnesium than sodium and calcium – in the right proportions – which helps push water and waste out of the cells
- High in all essential vitamins and minerals
- Low-fat food
- Good-quality protein

- Good-quality carbohydrate
- High in fibre
- Clean the gut
- Cleanse toxins from the body
- High in natural sodium

Food flushers

Fennel	Liver and digestion stimulant
Artichoke	Blood-sugar stabilizer
Dandelion	Natural diuretic
Dill	Anti-bloater
Carrots	Good all-rounder
Celery	High in natural sodium
Cucumber	Natural diuretic
Parsley	Natural diuretic
Beetroot	Detoxifies liver and gall bladder, cleans colon
Radishes	Stimulate gall bladder
Spinach	Shifts fluid retention
Watercress	Rich in *glucosinolates*, which help the liver detox
Red, Yellow & Orange Peppers	Betacarotene-rich
Nettles	Everything!
Lettuce	Contains silicon, which supports connective tissue
Cabbage, Broccoli, Brussels Sprouts, Kale & Cauliflower	All rich in glucosinolates
Tomatoes	High in bioflavonoids and lycopene
Asparagus	Natural diuretic
Avocado	High in lipase, a fat-busting enzyme
Chicory	Stimulates the liver
Alfalfa Sprouts etc	The most 'live' food you can find! Detoxifies.
Leeks	Natural diuretic

Fruit

Eating fruit also helps to remove excess sodium and acidity out of the cells and out of the body and, because *this* list of fruit is alkaline, it helps the body's pH balance as well. Fruit is 70–90 per cent made up of water with a very high sugar content. Natural, healthy sugar that gives you energy without the 'blood sugar blues'.

Fruit is also low in fat and high in fibre, which is very helpful for any healthy weight-loss programme, as well as a quick detox. These particular fruits are an extremely good source of vitamins and minerals. Cherries, blackcurrants and blackberries in particular are high in bioflavonoids – vitamin P – which is essential for strengthening capillaries and preventing fluid retention.

Fruit food flushers

Watermelon	Natural diuretic and cleanser
Strawberries	Lowest in natural fruit sugar, highest in vitamin C
Other Berries	Prevent fluid retention
Pineapple	Gut-cleaner and digestive enzyme
Apples	Help remove toxins and strengthen liver & digestion
Black Cherries	Prevent fluid retention
Citrus pith	Prevents fluid retention
Blackcurrants	Prevent fluid retention
Dark Grapes	Natural diuretic and good organ-cleansers
Peaches & Nectarines	Diuretic, cleansing and easily digested
Papaya & Mango	Gut-cleaner and digestive enzyme
Pink Grapefruit	Prevents fluid retention and supports liver
Apricots	Rich in potassium, help cells dump water
Figs	Rich in potassium, help cells dump water
Oranges & Tangerines	Help liver detox
Lemon	Makes the system alkaline, cleanses liver

Lime	Makes the system alkaline, cleanses liver
Kiwi	Contains natural digestive enzymes

An introduction to Omega 3 & 6 essential fatty acids

How EFAs help in weight loss

- Increase metabolism
- Fight fluid retention
- Suppress appetite
- Reduce cravings
- Increase energy
- Fill you up
- Make brain happy
- Help kidneys dump excess water

Hopefully, you've taken one look at this list and are now persuaded that essential fats are not fattening fats at all. In fact, essential fatty acids, Omega 3 and Omega 6, are so essential you can't lose weight without them! They increase your metabolism, heat production, and energy levels, which means that you burn more calories, even at rest. Although they are fats, they actually make it harder for your body to *make* fat and easier for it to burn fat.

Our bodies can't make these precious fats, so we have to get them from our food and most of us are getting nowhere near enough, *especially Omega 3*. Every single gland and organ in your body relies on EFAs for optimum health and if you want a healthy heart, joints and brain, as well as successful weight loss, think of EFAs as being as important for your body's health as calcium is for your bones.

EFAs help your kidneys to dump excess water held in your tissues – water that appears as extra weight. Essential fats also suppress your appetite and prevent carb and sweet cravings. They make you feel happier and lift depression, so you won't *want* to overeat. And they make you feel more like being physically active, so you burn even more calories. Convinced?

Omega 3-rich oils

Flaxseed oil, also known as linseed oil

Flaxseed oil is the richest source of the essential fatty acid most lacking in our diet: *Omega 3* (alpha-linolenic acid). It also contains small amounts of the other essential fatty acid we can't make for ourselves: Omega 6 (linoleic acid).

Hempseed oil

Dr Udo Erasmus, the world's leading expert on oils and author of the book *Fats that Heal, Fats that Kill*, considers hempseed oil to be nature's most perfectly balanced oil, due to its high content of *both* Omega 3 and Omega 6. And, despite its origins (the Cannabis sativa plant) it's completely legal and safe!

Omega 3 & 6 oil blend

To ensure a perfect balance of Omega 3 and 6, you can buy ready-blended oil, such as Udo's Choice. This is particularly recommended for the Slimmer's Smoothies weight-loss plan, when large quantities of oil will be consumed.

Recommended oils plan by plan

> **Kickstart detox:** flaxseed *and/or* hempseed oil *and/or* a blended oil
> **Long-term detox:** flaxseed *and/or* hempseed oil *and/or* a blended oil
> **Slimmer's smoothies:** blended oil, such as Udo's Choice
> **High-protein, low-carb:** flaxseed oil *or* hempseed oil *or* blended oil

Lecithin granules

These are a 'fat-loving' supplement a bit like washing-up liquid breaking down, or emulsifying, fats in the body. It is 57 per cent

Omega 6 to 7 per cent Omega 3, and is essential to have alongside flaxseed oil so you obtain the correct balance of Omega 3 and 6. It also turns any smoothie into a real milk shake, without the milk.

Unsalted nuts & seeds

Almonds, brazils, cashews, pecans, walnuts etc

Nuts, unsalted, are all rich in Essential Fatty Acids (Omega 3 and 6) which will help regulate your metabolism and therefore aid weight loss. A handful of nuts a day will also provide valuable protein and calcium.

Pumpkin, flax, sesame and sunflower seeds & pine nuts

All these little powerhouses of nutrition also provide a rich source of EFAs, protein and vitamins and minerals.

Protein

'Live' full-fat yoghurt – provides B vitamins and is richer in A and D than the milk from which it comes.

Quark – an extremely low-fat cheese

Cottage cheese – a low-fat cheese

Apart from nuts and seeds, which are an excellent source of protein, I've also incorporated a little dairy protein to help fight the flab. This may sound like a bit of a contradiction but there are four very good reasons why these proteins can help:

1 A LACK of protein, as well as an EXCESS of protein, can cause fluid retention because it prevents the liver from making enough albumin, which is ESSENTIAL for preventing fluid retention.

2 Protein is also needed to make hormones, such as thyroxin, the thyroid hormone that controls our metabolism.

3 When you mix one of the recommended oils with quark or cottage cheese, the amino acid cysteine in these proteins carries more energy and oxygen into your cells.

4 Recent research findings suggest that **lipase** could be a key enzyme for weight loss because it helps fat to be broken down properly instead of being stored in the fat cells. Lipase is found in all high-fat, 'live' foods such as **avocados, full-fat 'live' yoghurt, soaked seeds and nuts.**

Other foods to incorporate

Miso – Miso is made from fermented soybean paste and is rich in an alkaloid called dipicolonic acid, which helps drag toxins out of the body safely. You can find miso in an instant 'Cup-a-soup' form for your detox.

Sea vegetables – Dulse, Arame, Wakami and Nori are the richest source of organic mineral salts such as magnesium, potassium, calcium and sodium. They are also very rich in iodine, which is essential for the thyroid to regulate metabolism.

Garlic – a powerful detoxifier
Fresh Ginger – helps the liver detox
Turmeric – helps the liver detox

Drinks

2 litres of still water a day – drink at body temperature
Herbal teas – green tea, in particular, is full of toxin-fighting antioxidants.
Dandelion tea – helps to drain liver and gall bladder so great for a detox.

Nettle tea – stimulates the kidneys to release more water, naturally.
Detox teas – there are many containing detox helpers such as: liquorice, ginger, dandelion, fennel seeds, parsley and turmeric.
Miso instant soup – can be bought in sachets and usually contains sea vegetables so is an easy-to-prepare, detoxing hot drink.

Water

Water is the most important fluid to drink during a detox and also happens to be the world's best natural diuretic. You can still have as much of the recommended herbal teas as you like, but if you suffer from fluid retention it's probably because you don't drink enough water and your body's holding on to the little there is.

Water is the 'magic' ingredient when it comes to successful weight loss as well. It suppresses the appetite, fills you up and maintains blood-glucose levels by releasing sugar from the cells when needed, so cravings disappear. A lot of people lose weight *just* by drinking 2 litres of water a day.

When there is enough water in the body, the blood and lymphatic fluid can flow more easily. The blood takes enzymes and nutrients to the organs and the lymph fluid takes waste away to the elimination routes: skin, nose, bowel, kidneys and lungs. The more water you drink the more often you will use those elimination routes and the less waste and toxicity will be left in the body.

So that is your list of super foods for the 48-Hour Kickstart Detox. There are plenty of recipes incorporating many of the fruits and vegetables in chapter 13.

But first, let's Get Up and Go and discover *why* exercise is as essential as diet when it comes to losing weight.

6.

G – Get Up and Go

Hippocrates said, 'To rest is to rust, to rust is to decay.'

Well, nearly half of us *are* rusting because we're almost completely sedentary! Some of us spend half of every day watching TV, the rest is spent on the computer, on the phone, eating, talking to our friends, and basically sitting on our bums. And it's showing up on our scales with record levels of obesity in this country, even amongst the very young.

You CANNOT lose weight effectively if you don't exercise at least 4 times a week. I am living proof of this. It doesn't matter what or how little you eat, if you're not burning your food off, eventually you'll end up wearing it round your tummy and thighs. Sorry to be so blunt, but if you want to lose weight PERMANENTLY you need to say to yourself right now: I am going to build an hour's exercise into my day at least 4 times a week. Even if the only time I have is three 20-minute slots, I'm going to do it.

Regular exercise is ESSENTIAL if you want to lose real body fat. In just three months of regular exercise you could go down a whole dress size. But you may well have gained pounds of lean muscle tissue as well, so there is NO POINT WEIGHING YOURSELF. You will have become a lean, mean, calorie-burning machine – I promise.

The exercise I found that worked best for me, 'hot' yoga, changed my whole body shape, resulting in sculpted shoulders, muscle definition, a slimmer tummy (I'm still working at it!) and waist, and a drop in dress size. And that was after 4–5 sessions a week over just three months. I only lost a few pounds in weight, but I lost more than a few inches in flab. I built up the frequency slowly, starting with just a couple of sessions a week till my body got used to it. And I went for long, brisk walks in between. That is what worked for me. Everyone is different and you need to find what works for you.

Why you won't lose weight without exercise

The muscle mass of a 30-year-old is less than that of a 20-year-old. It's just a sad fact of life that if we're not working our muscles as we age we're going to lose muscle mass and without muscle mass our metabolism will slow down by between 2 and 5 per cent every 10 years. As I've already explained, that could mean an extra stone in weight by your mid-forties!

The good news is that by just putting on 3 lb of muscle mass you could *increase* your metabolism by as much as 7 per cent and lose that weight at the recommended 1–2 lb a week.

Don't worry, you don't need to hit the gym and start lifting dumbbells three times a week to achieve this. There are other ways to develop muscle mass without leaving your home, as you'll find out in chapter 13. And you won't need any additional equipment or special clothes.

Why exercise is good for you

Regular exercise isn't only essential for a healthy heart, bones and optimum weight. It's also essential for getting rid of toxicity. The skin is the largest elimination organ in the body and by sweating as often as possible, you'll be throwing those toxins out of your body on a regular basis.

A study carried out in America on more than five thousand healthy centenarians (100-year-olds) found they only had one thing in common. They worked up a good sweat every single day – running, chopping wood, making love, gardening, dancing and so on. Some smoked like chimneys, some drank, some ate red meat every day, others were vegetarians. But they ALL 'glowed' on a daily basis.

Exercise also makes you happy. After 20 minutes of working out (and brisk walking will do it) your body releases endorphins: 'feelgood' hormones that exercisers get addicted to. It's impossible to feel down in the dumps or in a bad mood after walking, dancing or working out for more than 20 minutes.

What type of exercise

For losing weight permanently, you need to do a combination of anaerobic and aerobic exercise.

Aerobic exercise

- Brisk Walking
- Jogging
- Swimming
- Steps
- Running
- Dancing
- Cycling
- Yoga (Ashtanga, Bikram, Hot or Dynamic)
- Tae-bo
- Kick-Boxing
- Circuit Training
- Spinning
- Rowing

Aerobic means 'requiring oxygen' and how efficiently the body gets that oxygen to the muscles. The stronger and healthier your heart, the more efficient your blood will be at getting oxygen to the muscles and the more aerobically fit you'll become. And the more aerobically fit you are, the more calories you burn – even at rest.

Anaerobic exercise

- Brisk Walking Carrying Weights
- Weight Training
- Resistance Training
- All Yoga (using your own limbs as weights)
- Uphill Walking

Anaerobic exercise requires less oxygen but requires muscular *strength*. Exercising your muscles, as in weight training, will burn calories faster than anything else. Using light weights, or your own limbs as weights, will develop lean tissue, and the more muscle you develop, the more you will burn calories. It will chisel and define your arms, legs, hips and bottom – and you won't look like a professional body builder one little bit!

How often, how long

The experts used to think that only aerobic exercise burned fat, but now, thanks to new research, we know that aerobic exercise COMBINED with weight training is the very best you can do for successful weight loss.

To reduce your body fat *radically* you need to do a minimum of 2–3 sessions a week of weight or resistance training PLUS 3 sessions a week of aerobic exercise. Or you can combine the two for a minimum of 4 times a week, advises Wayne Leonard, an exercise physiologist.

One of the best examples of combining aerobic and anaerobic exercise is power-walking and carrying weights, preferably uphill whenever possible! Wayne also recommends 'interval training', which means 2 minutes of very fast walking, followed by 1 minute of slow walking. This gets the heart rate to rapidly rise and drop, which will help you burn fat more effectively.

You could also combine aerobic and anaerobic exercise by finding a yoga class, like I did, that is both muscle-resistant and aerobic.

Some research shows that doing repeated bouts of exercise actually burns MORE calories than doing one prolonged session, because you are continually revving up your metabolism, which will stay revved up long after you've finished.

Others say you should be aiming for a minimum of 15 minutes and a maximum of 2 hours exercise a day. But it has to fit into your lifestyle, or you won't do it. If it suits you to exercise for 10 minutes in the morning, 10 minutes at lunchtime and 20 minutes in the evening, that's better than not doing it at all. Whatever you do, just make sure that you are **as active as possible, as often as possible.**

Example

If you get up from your desk for 1 minute **every hour** and run up and down the stairs, have a quick dance, or simply do a few stretching exercises, you will have done an extra 40 minutes over a week. Make it 2 minutes an hour and you will have accomplished nearly an hour and a half of physical exercise a week!

My two personal favourites for weight loss

Walking

Walking is a great way to start exercising. It won't wear out your joints to the same degree as other exercise, and it's what we're built to do. After all we walked for thousands of years till the wheel was invented. You don't need special training, clothes or equipment. You just need a good pair of walking shoes or trainers. You can walk anywhere, any time and you're never too old or unfit to begin, even if you only start with 5 minutes a day.

Studies of walkers who walk in excess of 5 mph (that's very fast) estimate that they burn *twice* as many calories as runners travelling at the same pace – because they are using more muscle power all over the whole body, using their arms to pump and taking longer strides. It is a more 'resistant' type of exercise than gentle jogging.

You don't need to walk that fast. Brisk walking is still an excellent way to shed excess pounds.

There will be a guide on how best to walk to burn fat in chapter 13, but if you are over 40 or have never exercised before, it might be an idea to check with your doctor first.

Dynamic or 'hot' yoga

This style of yoga is both aerobic and muscle-resistant. It is one of the best ways to lose weight and develop muscle tone, and you sweat. I have practised many different types of Hatha yoga over the years, but the Dynamic yoga I practise is the only type of yoga that has really made a difference to inches round my middle in a very short time. Previously I was only practising 1–2 times a week, this time I have been practising a *minimum* of 4–5 times a week, so the frequency may well have helped. I suspect that even if you followed the gentler Hatha every day, you would have much the same results, **as long as you are eating less than before.**

The benefits of all 'hot' yoga

Dynamic yoga is based on powerful deep breathing and heat. This style of yoga is derived and inspired by many different kinds of yoga, including Ashtanga. It is carried out in a heated room because, according to my teacher in Hove, Stuart Tranter, you are very unlikely to injure yourself if you have a very hot body. 'The hotter you become, the more elastic your muscles, ligaments and tendons become,' says Stuart. 'It's a bit like metal that's hard and cold and extremely strong, but when heated becomes pliable and bendy. This also promotes sweating, which will flush toxins out of your body on a regular basis.'

Heat also breaks down fatty tissue, working the body at a cellular level. The minimum temperature recommended is 75 degrees, but anyone wanting to try Bikram yoga, be warned – the room is exceptionally hot at 110 degrees.

Usually, according to Stuart, during aerobic exercise the body will start burning fat *after* 40 minutes. In a heated room, as the heart rate goes up and down it trains the body to use fat as a fuel almost immediately.

This, like ALL types of yoga, is a muscle-resistant exercise because you're using your own limbs as weights and counterweights. So you're carrying out weight training on your yoga mat with no equipment other than your own body.

I do the same series of postures every day; other yoga classes do different exercises each time. Whether you go for 'hot' yoga or any other yoga, find a class that you get on with and where the room is heated. Make sure it makes you sweat and raises your heart rate and you breathe deeply. And if it feels like 20 minutes, instead of the general one-and-a-half-hour discipline, you've found the right class.

If you've never exercised before, don't worry. In chapter 13 you will find a series of muscle-resistant exercises you can do at home, as well as advice on how to walk aerobically.

In the next chapter we explore less strenuous ways of losing fat and detoxing by looking at some of the holistic therapies available on the high street. I'm not suggesting you take yourself to the nearest beauty salon or health spa *instead* of exercising, but you might like to consider giving yourself an occasional treat in between your 4–5 sessions of fat-burning exercise a week or at the end of your detox.

7.

H – Holistic Therapies

Acupuncture – Acupuncture has been used in Chinese medicine for more than 3,000 years. Fine needles are inserted into certain acupoints in the body, which connect to 14 main channels, known as 'meridians'. Most of the meridians connect with a particular organ and this treatment helps to balance the flow of vital energy (qi) in the body. Apart from being used to treat dozens of conditions and ailments it can be very useful as part of a weight-loss programme to release toxicity, improve the function of your organs and your immune system, and to give you more energy.

Acupressure – Acupressure is like acupuncture without the needles. Using fingertip pressure on acupoints in the body, it can stimulate meridian flow and internal organ function and is very useful for releasing water retention and toxicity. You'll be learning your own facial acupressure exercises during your detox weekend, in chapter 13. There's more on this later in this chapter.

Aromatherapy – Essential oils are used to massage your muscles and help your blood and lymph to flow better. This can release toxicity and water retention and is very relaxing. You'll be learning how to use the oils yourself at home during your detox weekend, in chapter 13. See page 45 for more information.

Colonic hydrotherapy – Think of this as a total spring-clean of your colon! This treatment is recommended for the end of any detox, because it will help get rid of years of debris that the detox will have started shifting. Apart from anything else, it's one of the quickest ways to get that stomach even flatter. More later.

MLD – Manual lymphatic drainage is a very gentle massage, carried out by a therapist, which will stimulate the lymphatic system to drain and eliminate toxins from the body. A course is usually recommended to help with weight loss, alongside exercise and a healthy diet. It's a very relaxing treatment and is helpful for improving the appearance of cellulite.

Reflexology – Reflexology is based on the principle that various reflex points on the foot relate to the internal organs. The therapist uses his or her fingers and thumbs firmly, but gently, all over your feet, stimulating all the nerve endings. This allows energy to flow more freely; helping to break down congestion, clear toxicity, and restore harmony to the body, all the time completely relaxing you.

Seaweed wrap During a very relaxing hour and a bit, you will have your body exfoliated and massaged with aromatherapy oils, then a seaweed mask will be applied to your abdomen and thighs. You're then wrapped in a heated blanket to sweat all those toxins out! This is a fantastic 'quick fix' that can help you lose inches of water retention from all those areas where cellulite loves to hang out. A course is usually recommended for the best results.

These are just a few of the many holistic therapies you can try out to speed up inch loss, along with your new eating plan and exercise regime. Each one can help enormously but should be viewed as the icing on the cake. They can't replace a proper detox or a sensible diet. They can also cost a lot of money and take up a big chunk of your time.

But they are particularly useful during the lead-up to a special event or at the end of your detox. I heartily recommend that, provided you have the time and money, you look into what's on offer, have a good chat with the therapist and give one of them a try. If you have the time, but *don't* have the money, you could always try your local college to see if it needs 'guinea pigs' for its training courses. It could save you a fortune.

For the purposes of your 48-Hour Kickstart Detox we're going to concentrate on two of the therapies you can do yourself at home: facial acupressure and aromatherapy self-massage and baths. You will find details on how to do both in the privacy of your own home in chapter 13.

First, here is an explanation of how they work and why you should think about introducing them into your daily plan. I will also share my secrets with you on why I think colonic hydrotherapy is the ONE therapy well worth considering AFTER any major detox.

Aromatherapy oils

Aromatherapy oils are extracted from plants and are highly concentrated and powerful. The oils have many therapeutic components and, during a massage, help the blood and lymph to flow more freely, and if the lymph is working properly, those stubborn inches of water retention will come off all the more easily. Oils massaged into the skin pass through into the bloodstream and can then influence your entire body's health as well as your mental wellbeing.

As stress can inhibit all of the body's major functions, affecting circulation and lymphatic drainage, even *self*-massage, using the appropriate essential oils, can have a profound effect on you. At home, you can also make use of specific oils that target cellulite and water retention. Aromatherapist Vanessa Ough has come up with her list of suggested oils and how to use them for massage or in your bath in chapter 13, Kickstart Detox.

Acupressure

Much like acupuncture, dating back thousands of years, acupressure works on the flow of vital energy shown as qi, or chi, in the body. When this flow is blocked we can look puffy and water-retentive. The supply and flow of this vital energy, according to Chinese medicine, goes throughout the body along channels known as meridians, each one relating to a major organ.

One of the simplest techniques to stimulate the organs that need to let go of water is acupressure. Using fingertips, or a thumb, the therapist applies pressure at specific points on the body known as acupoints. This stimulates meridian flow to encourage the internal organs to function properly.

During your 48-Hour Kickstart Detox, you will learn a simple, quick, and effective facial using acupressure to energize and tone your skin and muscles and to get rid of any water retention that may have accumulated around your face.

Hopefully, you'll be able to incorporate this mini-facial workout into your daily routine in the bathroom.

Colonic hydrotherapy

There is such media interest in colonic hydrotherapy that it is now not unusual to see TV programmes about it, read articles featuring male reporters trying it and hear about the latest celebrity to be seen coming out of one of the many clinics that offer it. Colonic hydrotherapy has become nearly as 'normal' as going to have a bikini wax. There is no question that people's energy, weight and skin problems clear up after a couple of sessions and, however you feel about a two-inch pipe being shoved up your bottom, this is one treatment I would thoroughly recommend you have at the end of your weekend detox.

A healthy colon is essential for weight loss because when it's clogged up with years of unexpelled matter, toxicity sets in, causing bloating, lethargy, bad breath and skin problems. To produce a healthy colon, you need to follow a detox and give your lower intestine a good spring-clean a couple of times a year.

The colonic treatment usually takes no longer than an hour, and doesn't hurt at all; in fact many people fall asleep during the process. Using a six-inch length of plastic tubing and a tank full of water, the therapist flushes away any thing that has stuck to the colon and been there for a very long time.

A slight 'crampy' feeling may be experienced before a release but this is normal and nothing to worry about. The therapist massages your tummy as she or he fills and empties the colon with water. You can choose to watch your 'stuff' flow through the clear plastic tube or not. But the therapist will usually tell you when she or he spots mucus, undigested food or signs of Candida.

After a colonic, you'll feel much 'lighter', your bowel movements will improve, toxicity will have left your gut AND you'll have a flat tummy. I have one a couple of times a year, after a detox of at least a week, and no longer suffer from bloating – ever. Go on, be brave, and book one for the end of your detox!

Having had a look at which treatments can help move toxicity out of your body, let's now look at what toxins actually are and how we can avoid overloading our body with them in the first place.

8.

T – Toxicity

Toxins that make you fat

As you have already read, fat cells just 'love' toxins and stash them away like mad to help protect your organs. The more toxins you have, the bigger your fat cells and the more weight you tend to accumulate in areas such as your thighs, tummy and arms – cellulite to you and me.

Most practitioners, including myself, consider toxins to be anything that gets into the cells and causes an imbalance and, as we've seen, an imbalance at cellular level can encourage water retention and weight gain. In this context, toxins can be anything from chemicals to air pollution, from sugar to painkillers. A toxin doesn't necessarily have to be something 'poisonous'. Anything that we breathe in, ingest or touch could be considered toxic by our body if it's not recognized as a 'friend'. Even stress can be considered a toxin because of the effect of prolonged stress on the body.

The more unnatural the component, the more unlikely it is to match our own molecules and the more our cells will hang on to water to protect our organs. Too many toxins and the liver will use all its energy cleansing the body of what it sees as an enemy rather than kickstarting the body's metabolism to lose weight. So if you want to lose weight – lose the toxins!

Apart from essential medication, these are the toxins to consider eliminating as much as you can; no matter what weight-loss programme you plan to follow.

Toxins

- Pre-packaged food
- Fast food or takeaways
- Non-organic food
- Fizzy drinks
- Coffee or tea
- Alcohol
- Sugar
- Nicotine
- Prescription drugs
- Over-the-counter medicine
- Social drugs
- Stress

Pre-packaged food

If you needed reminding on why packaged and processed food and drink are full of toxins, consider this. One of Britain's leading food authorities, Dr Erik Millstone, from the science and technology research unit at Sussex University, estimates that no fewer than 3,850 additives are used in packaged food and drinks in the UK and the EU today. He has calculated that an average person on today's diet consumes four kilos of additives every year. (That could be **four kilos of extra fat** cells over a year!)

Fast food and takeaways

Although not as likely to be stashed full of additives, fast food and takeaways are still prone to being loaded with salt or sugar. Fast food is also short of fibre and enzymes and often fried. As this food is very hard to digest, it could well add to your toxic load because it stays in the colon far longer than home-cooked meals. The longer the food is in the colon, the more it begins to rot and produce toxins – toxins which get absorbed into the bloodstream and taken to every cell in the body.

Non-organic food

'Eating non-organic produce is like taking part in a long-term experiment, swallowing something like *one gallon* of pesticides and organophosphates a year,' warns Roz Kadir, a nutritionist who specializes in performance-related nutrition. So that's another gallon of toxicity that could be hanging around the body stored in fat cells in the form of the chemical pesticides, herbicides and fungicides sprayed on non-organic crops.

Not only that, but non-organically reared animals are more likely to have been fed hormones, antibiotics or to have eaten grass contaminated by pesticides. These could all be passed to you in milk, cheese and meat, adding a few more pounds of extra toxins over the years.

● Fizzy drinks

High-calorie drinks are full of sugar which, although not strictly speaking a toxin, will raise blood-sugar levels, increase insulin production and turn you into a fat-producing machine if you don't burn it off. More importantly, both 'full fat' soft drinks as well as low-calorie drinks often contain additives and colourings such as formaldehyde, aspartic acid and phenylaline. These are all considered to be toxins by the liver, so they will get stored in your fat cells along with all the others.

● Coffee or tea
● Alcohol
● Sugar and sugary snacks

Stressed-out people who live off coffee, tea, alcohol and sugary snacks need to know that this will encourage their bodies to store more fat. When the adrenals are overworked (as with constant stress and stressful stimulants) they over-produce cortisol and insulin, which eventually causes water retention and fat storage – usually in the abdominal region.

A diet high in sugar also allows bad bowel bacteria to take over, upsetting the important acid/alkaline balance in the body, which can lead to a whole host of problems from bloating to Candida. Artificial sweeteners should be considered even more of a toxin, as they are artificially produced chemicals and will, inevitably, end up being stored in your fat cells.

● *Nicotine*

Smoking is obviously a toxin. Cigarettes contain thousands of toxic chemicals in the smoke and tar. Remember, all poisons that harm us, including the benzopyrin in cigarettes, are stored in the fat cells.

Nicotine replacement products may well wean you off the weed, but they too, along with ordinary chewing gum, should be considered toxins for the entirety of any detox or weight-loss plan. They will only encourage the body to hang on to water to protect the liver and other organs from all the chemicals they contain.

● *Prescription drugs*
● *Over-the-counter medicine*
● *Social drugs*

If you have to take a lot of medication over a long time (especially antibiotics) this will encourage an over-growth of acidity in the gut which can lead to Candida – and more bloating. You obviously shouldn't stop taking any essential medication, but it's worth considering what is deemed to be essential and what isn't, for the sake of your fat cells.

Even over-the-counter headache pills should be considered toxins if taken regularly. Dr Simon Ellis, consultant neurologist at North Staffordshire Hospital, says that if you are taking bought painkillers on more than seven days every month it's excessive for the liver's health. And you want a healthy liver if you're going to shift that weight.

Any social drug contains toxic chemicals so, again, do without them during your detox and as much as possible while you're on one of the weight-loss plans.

● *Stress*

It may seem strange to claim stress is a toxin but, as far as the body's concerned, it is. Nowadays most of us suffer from prolonged stress and that, combined with an excess of sugar and stimulants, causes the body to store more fat.

Stress stimulates the adrenals to produce 'fight or flight' hormones (adrenaline) by releasing sugar stores and raising blood-sugar levels to give our muscles and brain a boost of energy. But, because 21st-century stress is mainly mental and emotional and we're not fighting sabre-toothed tigers any more, that boost of energy has nowhere to go and the body stores the excess glucose as fat.

As well as affecting every cell in our body, stress affects our digestion – big-time. Everytime we get stressed, because the train is late or someone's cut us up in the fast lane, valuable blood is shunted away from our brain and intestines to our muscles to deal with the stress and we stop digesting our food properly. All that stress stays in our body, affecting our gut. This causes food intolerances, digestive disorders and a toxic build-up, which can account for pounds of excess weight in the form of undigested food and water retention.

During your 48-Hour Kickstart Detox, chapter 13, you'll have the opportunity to try out some exercises and techniques to help you relax and lead a more stress-free life.

So as you've seen, it's almost impossible to achieve a perfect metabolism if toxins and stress constantly bombard your body. If you're going to lose weight successfully, ANYTHING that causes stress, including stress itself, whether ingested as in coffee, cigarettes, alcohol, and sugar, or from the environment as in pesticides, additives, and chemicals, needs to be eliminated as much as possible to help you shrink those fat cells.

When it comes to toxins, the liver rules OK? In the next chapter we look at *how* the liver removes toxins from your body and how looking after your liver can help you lose weight.

9.
L – Liver

As you've read in the previous chapter, our bodies are constantly bombarded by toxins and it is the liver, the 'chemical factory', that has to deal with each and every one of them. Every single minute, more than a litre of blood passes through the liver so it can filter and remove bacteria and toxins from the circulation, making sure they're eliminated from the body.

From alcohol to pesticides, hormones and preservatives, even the chlorine in the tap water you drink, the liver has to make sure its enemies are destroyed and don't hang about in your body disrupting the balance of your cells. Your health, energy and ability to lose weight all depend on the health of your liver.

The liver holds the key to successful weight loss because it also plays a major part in your metabolism and to detox it will help it do its job properly so you will lose weight more easily and be able to move fat out of the body. If your liver is functioning properly you don't need to count calories, weigh food, go on a fast or feel hungry.

But a poor diet and lifestyle can cause excess stress to the liver, along with stress itself, and if your liver is stressed it won't do its job efficiently and you won't lose weight easily. This list shows just a few of the liver's enemies – the things that stress it out.

Liver foes

- Stress
- Caffeine
- Alcohol
- Drugs – prescription, social and over-the-counter drugs
- Exhaust and Paint Fumes
- High-Protein Diets
- Saturated Fats
- Hot Spices
- Sugar
- Chocolate

- The Pill
- HRT
- Cigarette Smoke

- Dehydration
- Watching TV for More than a Couple of Hours!

The liver as a fat-buster

The liver secretes a litre of bile a day, which acts much like a mild detergent emulsifying fatty acids so they can be absorbed. Bile is sent to the intestines, via the gall bladder, where it is absorbed by fibre and faeces and then excreted. Bile also helps increase peristaltic movement (bowel movements) so that waste is eliminated from the body as quickly as possible rather than sitting in your intestines rotting.

The liver and metabolism

The liver's health is also very important for proper protein-, fat- and, most importantly in regard to weight loss, carbohydrate metabolism. Carbs – in the form of sugars and starches – are broken down by the digestion and absorbed into the bloodstream. The blood then circulates round the body to the liver, where the sugars are converted into glucose, the fuel the body needs for energy.

A healthy liver regulates the use of glucose and allows certain levels to circulate in the blood for the cells to use when they need it. A sluggish liver will have more problems controlling the glucose release and your blood-sugar levels will become more unstable, causing cravings and binges.

The liver and water retention

The liver also breaks down aldosterone, an adrenal hormone that helps the kidneys to regulate salt and water balance. *Excessive* aldosterone production causes water and sodium retention – so you need the liver to be doing the best job it can to break it down.

Why detox

You know yourself when your liver's overloaded. If you've eaten too much rich food, and drunk too much alcohol, the liver becomes swollen and sluggish as it attempts to break it all down so it can recycle some of it and dispose of the rest. The next day you feel 'liverish' and your skin erupts with spots, your head thumps and you're bloated. All signs that there are too many toxins for your liver to deal with and that it needs a rest.

Signs of a liver in need of a detox!

• Dark Circles under Eyes	• Constipation
• Spots	• IBS
• Itchy Skin	• Fluid Retention
• Age Spots	• Headaches
• Sallow Skin	• Foggy Brain
• Poor Digestion	• Allergies
• Bloating	• Hot Palms or Feet
• Weight Gain around Abdomen	• Unstable Blood-sugar Levels

How the liver detoxes

The liver clears 99 per cent of all bacteria and toxins from the blood BEFORE it enters general circulation. But toxins need to be altered *chemically* before they can be excreted. They're not usually very soluble. The liver alters the toxins to become soluble so they can be taken safely out of the body via the colon and kidneys. It does this in two phases.

The liver needs to be supported throughout Phase 1 and 2 if it's going to do its job properly and without the myriad of detoxing symptoms normally associated with a cleanse.

Phase 1

The first phase is called oxidation, when toxins, hormones and other chemicals that your own body produces during a detox are attacked. Phase 1 enzymes either neutralize these, or break them down into other forms, which are then processed by Phase 2 enzymes. Each toxin is transformed by a chemical alteration into a less toxic form. As the liver's immune cells get to work on these toxins they release powerful inflammatory chemicals called free radicals, which need to be mopped up by antioxidants. If they're not mopped up properly, toxins are released back into the bloodstream, causing uncomfortable symptoms all over your body.

Phase 2

Phase 2 is another kind of alteration, called 'conjugation'. Each toxin is linked to another harmless substance so it can be made water soluble to be carried out of the body safely, via the colon and kidneys.

The liver needs to be supported by amino acids and certain properties found in food to be able to complete this stage. Otherwise, the toxins can accumulate in the fatty tissues, brain and all over your body, making you feel pretty rough.

You will read more about the supplements that best support the liver's two phases in chapter 12, Supplements.

The liver can completely regenerate itself in just 6 weeks, even if it's lost up to 90 per cent of its structure. It can still rebuild itself as a functioning organ, given the right foods. So if you can, try and follow the detox plan for longer than just 2 days – your liver will thank you for it and repay you with permanent weight loss and improved health and energy.

In the next chapter we look at water retention, or oedema. What it is and what causes it and how we're going to get rid of it in just 48 hours.

10.

O – Oedema: Water Retention

Strictly speaking, oedema is a medical condition based on heart and kidney weakness. But a milder form of oedema, or water retention, is something most women experience just before a period when as much as 7 lb in weight can suddenly appear on the scales out of nowhere. As you'll see, there are many other reasons why our bodies choose to hold on to water. The good news is that fluid retention can be eliminated in as little as 48 hours, if you first eliminate the cause.

What is oedema?

Fluid retention, or oedema, is just an excess of water in the body's tissues. Our cells are, for various reasons, saving water for an emergency and, as they swell, new water and nutrients can't get in. Unabsorbed water and nutrients then accumulate in the connective tissues surrounding the cells, causing swelling and water retention in the legs, kidneys, under the chin and in the fingers. We've become big swollen bags of water with fluid trapped in between the body's cells instead of being excreted by the kidneys. How many times can you not get your rings off at the end of the day?

Here are a few of the many reasons why our bodies hang on to water.

Dehydration

The body will hold on to excess water if you don't drink enough. When you are dehydrated, your body excretes less water, holds on to the little that's left in case of an emergency, and bloating sets in.

Constipation

If your colon isn't getting rid of waste once a day (preferably twice) your body is likely to retain fluid to dilute the partially digested foods still stuck in your gut. Again, the more water you drink, the more your colon will get rid of waste and the less you'll hang on to water.

EFA deficiency

Essential fatty acids are needed to produce hormone-like substances called prostaglandins. These control hormones and the balance of water throughout the menstrual cycle. Too few EFAs and the body is more likely to retain excess fluid in a last-ditch effort to produce prostaglandins.

Sugar & carbohydrate excess

Eating a lot of starch and sugar can make you heavy and bloated because every unit of glycogen produced from carbohydrate sugars is put aside by the body for energy. It needs three times as much water with which to store it. So the more starch and sugar you eat, the more water needs to be mobilized to convert the starches and sugars to glycogen. And the more waterlogged you become.

Sodium excess

Two of the most important minerals the body needs to regulate fluids are sodium and potassium. (The other two are calcium and magnesium.) But most of us have far too much sodium in our system and not nearly enough potassium, and this will induce fluid retention big-time.

An excess of sodium also forces the body to hold on to extra amounts of water to dilute the extra salt, and the tissues become waterlogged.

Allergies

Intolerances and allergies cause a sudden fluctuation in blood-sugar levels, which can lead to water retention. The most common offenders are: wheat, milk, eggs, yeast, sugar, food additives and nuts. Apart from nuts, all these foods will be eliminated during the 48-Hour Detox. Obviously, if you have a nut allergy, you will steer clear of those as well.

Hormones

Water retention can also be caused by hormone imbalances. From birth control pills to HRT, to pregnancy and the menopause, they can all contribute to hormonal havoc and fluid retention as your body frantically tries to balance.

Vitamin B6 plays an important role in the body's use of hormones associated with fluid retention in women. B6 helps the liver to metabolize hormones such as oestrogen and progesterone and so will help the body remove the water retention associated with PMT. It also helps the kidneys eliminate waste.

All the foods that are going to help you shift water retention are listed in chapter 13, the 48-Hour Kickstart Detox. They include natural diuretics, potassium-rich fruit and vegetables and foods high in B6 and EFAs.

11.

S – Synergy

Synergy or synergism means 'the working together of two or more components to be more successful or productive as a result of a merger'. In other words, you need more than two components in order to lose weight successfully. We've explored the use of the right foods, we've looked at which exercises will help, now we need to look at a third component. Something else that may help shift weight at a much deeper level – the emotional level: the link between the mind and the body.

Metaphysical counsellor Louise Hay, author of *You Can Heal Your Life*, believes that when there is weight gain and fluid retention there's often an emotional reason for putting on the pounds. When *she* feels insecure and ill at ease, she says, she puts on a few pounds. When the threat has gone, the excess weight goes away by itself. I tend to agree. Have you ever noticed how you can suddenly look pounds heavier just before a trip away that is stressing you out? She reckons the power of our own mind is the best diet she knows of. Go on a diet of negative thoughts and the weight will pile on. When we really love ourselves, everything else in our life works – including weight loss.

I have found this to be true of myself. If I look in the mirror and say, 'God, my thighs are getting thinner, this yoga's really working,' they really do look slimmer and other people start noticing. If I go through a 'fat' spell (and who doesn't?) and start saying, 'God, my thighs look fat and wobbly,' my whole body looks fatter and more wobbly and, although the inches may well be coming off, I don't LOOK or feel any better. The mind/body connection is VERY strong.

To get that mind/body connection working for you and your weight loss, we're going to look at four different synergies to help you change your mind-set. In chapter 13, 48-Hour Kickstart Detox, there will be some exercises that you can try out yourself in the privacy of your own home.

- T'ai Chi
- Affirmations
- Visualization
- Meditation

All of these techniques will make you feel more positive and help still your mind. They will make you feel happier, calmer and energized so you WANT to continue to lose weight.

They're going to help change your negative thoughts and energies to positive thoughts and energies. And they're going to help balance your Yin with your Yang for perfect harmony and balance.

T'ai Chi Ch'uan

The Chinese art of T'ai Chi Ch'uan has been around for more than 10 thousand years. It is a series of moves put together to create harmony for the mind, body and spirit. It is a moving meditation, a powerful tool for relaxation, as well as self-defence. It can also increase focus, concentration and clarity of mind, which are all very important for developing a positive attitude towards losing weight.

Regular practice allows the chi, or energy, to flow and circulate throughout the whole body and can help manage your weight by improving your posture, self-esteem and metabolic rate.

Penny May, a teacher in T'ai Chi Ch'uan, practises the original style of T'ai Chi, which includes Chi Kung. 'Without doubt, T'ai Chi Ch'uan brings your body to its natural weight through continual practice, although this is a side effect and not the main reason for doing T'ai Chi Ch'uan,' she says.

There is further information on where to find out more about T'ai Chi under references at the back of the book.

Affirmations & positive thinking

If indeed every thought we think is creating our future, then you need to change any negative thoughts into positive ones from now on! You need to change every thought about the past or the future into the *present*.

You need to *think* in the positive and in the present by saying things like, 'I now accept a wonderful slim body,' instead of 'I hate my body' or 'I want to have a slimmer body.' If you constantly say something in the future tense: I want, I wish for . . . etc, then it will stay there – *in the future*, that's how obedient our subconscious mind is. But say it in the present and it becomes the now.

We also need to love and approve of ourselves, trusting in the process of life and actually *believing* in the power of our own mind. I know it all sounds very wacky, but I promise you it really, really works.

I was a cynical, freelance journalist for years, always worrying about money and where the next job was coming from. As soon as I learned to trust that the Universe would provide and to stop worrying and being attached to the negative thought, the energy changed and a job or money always flowed in whenever I needed and *trusted* that it would be delivered – and it still does. (The Universe is just my thing, you can believe in whatever powers you like: God, Mohammed, Buddha, Self etc.)

It's the same with weight. If you truly believe that the Universe, or whatever, will give you what you need, including weight loss, IT WILL!

Visualization

How does a thought defeat a cancer cell? This is what I wrote about the link between mind and body in my last book:

'Very recently scientists found a nerve cell communicating with an immune cell – a lymphocyte – in a petri dish in a lab. For the first time scientists accepted what complementary therapists have believed for years. There *is* a link between the brain – and emotions

– and the immune system. This, they deduced, would affect the way lymphocytes behave and Psycho Neuro Immunology (PNI) was born. Psycho Neuro Immunology means "a bridge between psychology and the nervous and immune systems".

Dr Candace Pert, a leading PNI authority, says, 'Consciousness changes can create physical molecules in the body. This is a recent scientific finding and is as important as discovering the earth was round!'

No one is absolutely sure how it all works and most doctors are still very cynical about it. But these types of visualization exercises are being used more and more by cancer patients, with some success. And if it works for life-threatening diseases it must certainly be worth trying for dispersing a few fat cells.

You will find a useful visualization exercise I learned while attending a PNI course at the Bristol Cancer Help Centre in chapter 13.

Meditation

While visualizing every day is thought of as a form of 'watching', meditation is thought of as a form of 'witnessing' and is equally useful for a successful weight-loss programme.

The benefits of meditation have been verified in study after study. Millions of people around the world can testify to the positive effects of this practice. It calms and relaxes, rests and rejuvenates, produces a more positive outlook and reduces stress.

And, as you've seen, stress is one of the major contributors to unexplained weight gain or bloating.

By practising meditation you learn to quieten and still the mind. To see thoughts, however negative, plop into your mind but be able to ignore them and let them drift off again. The more you practise it the quieter your thoughts become. Eventually your mind will settle down completely, allowing you to get into the lovely tranquil state that babies and children naturally inhabit.

You don't need to sit cross-legged on the floor for 2 hours a day. Even if it's only 5 minutes, meditating regularly will reduce stress and fatigue, and really improve your chances of developing positive energy so the weight just falls off. You can find out more about learning to meditate in Resources.

In the next chapter we take a look at some of the supplements that can help you carry out a really successful detox, however short.

12.

S – Supplements for the Kickstart Detox

There are just three supplements you might want to consider taking during your detox. They're the best I've come across for helping the liver and colon to cleanse properly and they all help reduce many of the common side effects associated with detoxification, such as constipation, spots and headaches. They're not compulsory but I, personally, find these three so beneficial that I put them into my daily smoothie most days and not only during a detox. (There will also be one recommended supplement at the end of each of the subsequent 3 weight-loss plans, specifically chosen for the programme you're following.)

48-Hour Detox supplements

- Milk Thistle
- Lecithin
- Colon Cleanser

Why supplements help a detox

Nutritionist Dr Lawrence Plaskett, Principal of Plaskett Nutritional Medicine College, is, like many other experts, aware that the original idea of fasting to promote health or weight loss doesn't really work. That's because detoxification needs certain nutrients, such as antioxidants, if the toxins are to be taken out of the body safely. As explained in chapter 9 on the liver, toxins need to be altered chemically before they can be excreted safely. Otherwise, according to Dr Plaskett, the tissues are loaded with toxic substances, the metabolic processes of the body slow down, affecting energy, vitality and enzyme production, and instead of feeling light and clean you end up feeling even more toxic and sluggish.

In order to kickstart your system for a successful detox and weight-loss programme, the liver needs all the help it can get to alter the toxins and send them on their way out of the body, via the bowel, safely and quickly. And there isn't a better supplement to support the liver in this process than milk thistle.

Milk thistle

Milk thistle has been used as a traditional liver tonic for centuries to heal, protect and regenerate the liver. It is a member of the daisy family, known as silybum marianum, and is renowned for its ability to protect the liver from damage and stimulate new, healthy cells. It has even been found to speed up recovery from jaundice and to protect against hepatitis and cirrhosis.

On a day-to-day basis, it will protect your liver from alcohol and prescription drugs, without affecting the medicine's effectiveness and potency. So this is a wonderful herb to keep permanently in your cupboard to take the morning after the night before!

Milk thistle is also a potent antioxidant and increases the amount of *glutathione* in the liver – a powerful tool for cleansing. As far as the detox goes, this is the liver's main antioxidant for mopping up free radicals produced by toxins. Without it, the mopping-up process may not be as successful as it could be and toxins could end up back in the bloodstream, causing uncomfortable symptoms all over the body.

So you can see why I think this is a very helpful supplement to take during a detox, during party season or when you're simply feeling under the weather.

You might like to take another look at the list of symptoms associated with a sluggish liver, because all of them can be treated quite safely using milk thistle, especially skin disorders. Because it also increases your liver's ability to break down dietary fats, your bowel will work better and you'll feel more energetic when you add this supplement to your regime – especially during a detox.

Conditions that milk thistle can help

- Alcohol Excess
- Drug Excess
- Spots
- Itchy Skin
- Bloating
- Fluid Retention
- Headaches
- Foggy Brain
- Allergies
- Unstable Blood-sugar Levels
- Feeling Under the Weather

Lecithin granules

The name 'lecithin' is derived from the Greek word for egg yolk, from which it was first produced. It is now usually made from soybean oil, so is high in essential fatty acids – Omega 3 and, in particular, Omega 6.

Lecithin has been hailed for its ability to prevent sticky artery walls as well as reducing cholesterol and protecting and regenerating the liver. Because of its high choline (vitamin B) content, it is also wonderful for the brain's health and for improving memory – as well as helping you to feel a little sharper after a heavy night.

When you combine lecithin granules with essential fats in a smoothie, the lecithin breaks down the oils, turning the smoothie into a creamy milk shake without the milk. You'll find this wonderful stuff recommended to add to both the detox smoothies, in chapter 13, and the Slimmer's Smoothies in chapter 15.

Colon cleanser

Psyllium husks plus probiotics and pre-biotics

Fibre is essential for detoxing and losing weight because it helps to get the colon moving, getting the toxicity released out of the body as quickly as possible. It is like a broom sweeping your intestines clean. If you add pre-biotics and probiotics to the fibre, you have a supplement that will not only clean your gut, but will also make sure your good bacteria positively proliferate! By providing natural fibre and friendly bacteria to work together you will be blessed with optimum colon performance, which can only mean one thing: no more bloating.

These are the three components that should be included in any natural fibre powder you buy to encourage regular bowel movements and the release of toxins.

Fibre – psyllium husks

Made from the husks of an Indian plant's seeds, psyllium is high in natural fibre. When mixed with fluid, this *soluble* fibre acts like a sponge, absorbing more than twenty times its weight to form a soft gel or mucilage. This will help remove months of undigested matter, toxicity and debris from your gut to be eliminated safely.

Fibre is an essential part of any detox because mucilage, or soluble fibre, takes cholesterol, bile acids and toxicity out of the body, making sure you are eliminating waste regularly. This ensures a healthy bowel movement *twice* a day, no matter what or how little you might be eating. This type of fibre also stabilizes blood-sugar levels as it slows down the amount of glucose produced, therefore avoiding those fluctuating blood-sugar highs and lows.

Pre-biotics

Pre-biotic means 'relating to living organisms or produced by the action of living organisms': healthy bacteria. We used to get plenty of pre-biotics from the soil our vegetables were grown in. But our food is so clean, washed and packaged in plastic nowadays that there is very little left.

The most important pre-biotic is FOS – fructo oligosaccharides. Oligo means 'few' and saccharide means 'sugar'. Oligosaccharides can only be partially broken down by your digestive system, so when they are consumed the undigested part becomes *a food* for the probiotics (the friendly guys) in your gut, so they can get nice and strong and healthy!

Probiotics

Probiotics are friendly bacteria needed to keep your intestinal bacteria healthy. If unfriendly bacteria take over, bloating, gas and more serious health problems such as Candida, chronic fatigue and IBS can develop.

But if you have more good bacteria than bad, the good will break down the fibre and waste in your colon and get everything moving out as well as keeping the bad guys at bay.

Lactobacillus acidophilus and Bifidobacterium bifidum are two of the most important natural probiotics to look for in any colon cleanser. On a day-to-day basis, they will also help improve bowel conditions such as IBS and colitis, as well as protecting the health of your colon after a course of antibiotics or prolonged stress. These two probiotics are very well known for their ability to help prevent travellers' tummy and are usually found in foods such as 'live' or 'bio' yoghurt.

All three of these colon helpers – psyllium husks, pre-biotics and probiotics – can be found in various colon powders.

So that's your Top Three supplements for a successful detox – the detox you're about to embark on!

The next chapter is the one we've been building up to for the last twelve chapters – your Kickstart Detox Weekend. Are you ready? This is it, 48 Hours to Kickstart Healthy Weight Loss, using the next two days to lose as much fluid retention as you can and come out the other end (excuse the pun) with a flatter stomach, a calmer mind and a whole new positive attitude to weight loss.

13.

Kickstart Detox

Welcome to the 48-Hour Kickstart Detox: your two days to relax, recuperate, rejuvenate and lose inches of fluid retention. If you haven't read the previous chapters, don't worry – you can start *planning* for your detox now. But don't just go ahead and give up everything you're used to eating and drinking without preparing first. As I said before, you can't give up all your favourite 'poisons' at the same time or you'll end up feeling terrible and wishing you had never started.

You'll also need to stock up on food and other essentials to make your weekend an enjoyable experience: more of a health spa than a health farm! So please take the time to read through this chapter to see which techniques you're going to experiment with, what recipes appeal to you and, most important of all, how long you need as a countdown to the big day. Prepare well ahead of time, and you'll fly through the weekend without any of the side effects so often associated with detoxification.

And please don't forget, even if you want to go straight to one of the three weight-loss plans that follow this chapter, you will lose weight more quickly and successfully if you kickstart your body with a detox first.

Countdown to detox – eliminate or cut down:

Four weeks:	Fried food, ready-made meals, chemicals & painkillers
Two weeks:	Alcohol, wheat, coffee, sugar and salt
One week:	Red meat, potatoes, and dairy products

Try and plan your Kickstart weekend for a few weeks ahead, when you know you can lock the door and hide away without any interruptions or temptations. Don't leave it till the last minute and eliminate all of the above in one week, or you'll need painkillers and alcohol to get through it!

Whatever your particular 'addiction' is, cut down gradually. For example, if you always have two big glasses of wine a night:

Week 1	Halve the amount – one glass a night
Week 2	Halve the intake again – one very small glass a night
Week 3	Halve again – one small glass every other night
Week 4	Try and have it once or twice a week only

Work out your own plan, with your own diary and work out something that really works for you and you alone. Or do it with a friend so you can encourage and support each other and even compete with each other!

From now on, take the following lists everywhere with you. If you want to know more about why you are eliminating these things, read chapter 4 – Eliminate. Suffice to say that these are the very substances that encourage your body to hold on to water quicker than anything else. Detoxification clears stuff like this from the body by neutralizing it and transforming it into waste and water, so the more weight you'll lose – albeit fluid excess rather than fat.

Cut down on the following in this order of priority:

- Over-the-Counter Drugs
- Recreational Drugs
- Tobacco
- Fried Food
- Crisps
- Ready-Made Meals
- Cakes and Pastries
- Soft Drinks
- Chocolates & Sweets
- Alcohol
- Wheat & Pasta
- Coffee
- Red Meat
- Potatoes
- Dairy Products
- Tea

Cut down on these animal products in this order of priority:

- Sausages, Bacon & Processed Meats
- Offal
- Pork
- Beef
- Lamb
- Dairy
- Eggs
- Poultry
- Chicken or Game
- White Fish
- Oily Fish

In the last week leading up to your Kickstart Detox, give your liver the best proteins to help it cleanse: baked beans, pulses such as hummus, seeds, unsalted nuts (*not* peanuts), a little fish and chicken, brown basmati rice and lots of fresh fruit, steamed vegetables and salads.

But the most important thing you need to do from now on, if you do nothing else, is to start drinking more water, building up to 2 litres a day. Start drinking a small glass of still water every hour on the hour and you'll soon be consuming 2 litres. It will help keep your blood-sugar levels even, prevent cravings and fill you up. You'll also look better and have more energy – promise!

Drink one glass of water for every coffee or tea you have but don't beat yourself up if you can't get through a busy day without your cuppa. If you find it really hard to function and you're getting headaches, make it *one* freshly ground, organic, black tea or coffee a day – even during the detox. I want you to sail through your weekend, not suffer from horrible side effects. (The only de-caf I would recommend is water-treated and therefore chemical-free.)

These are some of the detox symptoms you might experience if you give up too much, too soon. Hopefully you'll take it really gently, but should the worst happen:

Detox symptoms & solutions

Constipation: Drink more water and eat dried fruit such as prunes or apricots.

Bloating: Hot water with a slice of lemon; dill or fennel tea.

Spots: Dab on tea tree essential oil. Drink more water.

Headache: A product called '4-Head' is completely natural and on sale in pharmacies and supermarkets.

Wind: Camomile, dill, fennel or peppermint tea or warm vinegar with a little honey.

Insomnia: Camomile tea, a few drops of lavender oil on the pillow (don't let it get near your eyes), Valerian tincture drops, or a *cold*-water footbath.

Nausea: Fennel or peppermint tea, ginger tea, and barley water.

Cold sores: A few drops of undiluted lemon juice, or Melissa essential oil, two or three times a day.

Colds: Take a vitamin C supplement with added zinc. Consult a pharmacist for dosage.

So that's the bad news, now for the good. The Kickstart Detox is going to encourage your cells to let go of inches of water retention, bloating and toxicity as quickly as possible – but they need the best tools for the job, a 10-point plan:

On the kickstart weight-loss detox you will

1. Drink at least 2 litres of water a day
2. Eat water-based foods to flush the kidneys
3. Improve enzyme & liver function by eating raw
4. Eat more 'live' food
5. Choose organic wherever possible
6. Sweat those toxins out
7. Boost your metabolic rate
8. Clean your 'guttering'
9. Eat the right amount, at the right time
10. Switch the outside world off

Drink at least 2 litres of water a day

Water is magic when it comes to a successful detox and weight loss: it suppresses your appetite, clears waste and toxicity, helps your bowels move AND, as it's nature's very own diuretic, water gets rid of water retention!

Once you're drinking enough (your urine should be 'straw'-coloured and your eyes will look brighter), bloating and fluid retention will be a thing of the past.

> **! TOP TIPS** MAKE SURE YOUR WATER IS:
>
> Still, Not Fizzy
> Room-Temperature
> Mineral or Filtered
> Not Drunk *with* Meals – leave at least 30 minutes either side of a meal
> Not Drunk After 9.00 p.m.
> Not Exceeding 2 Pints in One Go

Hot drinks

You can make up your 2 litres of water a day with hot drinks and natural fluid eliminators such as: dandelion, nettle or detox tea. If you're missing your caffeine fix, green tea is a good substitute as it contains a little **natural** caffeine. But if you're really struggling, you can have one cup of organic, black tea or coffee a day.

Another hot drink that will really get those cells detoxing, fill you up and warm you up is miso. Miso is made from fermented soybean paste and helps produce healthy intestinal flora. It is also rich in dipicolonic acid, which will literally link on to toxins in your body and drag them out. You can buy 'Cup-a-soup'-type miso broth in most health stores.

Eat water-based foods to flush the kidneys

The foods on your shopping list (see page 85) are high-alkaline foods, natural diuretics, rich in flavonoids, water, and essential minerals that encourage the body to excrete sodium and water.

As the Kickstart Detox only lasts for 2 days, I urge you, in the words of Mahatma Gandhi, to 'eat your drinks and drink your food'. In other words, make as many of your meals as possible liquid meals, such as smoothies, juices and soups. The less energy the body needs to digest food, the more energy it will have to cleanse and the more inches of fluid retention you'll lose. The more watery your meals, the more water you'll lose!

During your Kickstart Detox, you may find that you spend more time on the loo at night weeing. This is a very good sign that the sodium (and therefore the water retention) is moving out of your cells and out of your body.

Improve enzyme & liver function by eating raw

It's been found that animals fed on cooked diets always weigh more than animals on raw-food diets, even if the calorie intake is equal. Dr Howell at the Lindlahr Sanatorium also noticed that it's impossible for people to gain weight on enzyme-rich raw foods, regardless of the calories.

Enzymes are essential for breaking down and digesting food, but if the environment is too acid, as opposed to alkaline, the enzymes don't work very well and undigested food ends up dumped in the colon, rotting and causing bloating.

Enzymes also help the body repair and maintain itself and are believed, by some, to help us stay young!

Eat more 'live' food

You can't get more 'live' than sprouted beans and seeds. They possess all the energy, goodness and power that enable them to grow from a tiny seed to a strong, fully grown plant – packed full of enzymes, minerals and vitamins. If you want energy (and you *need* energy to lose weight!) eat your sprouts.

I used to hate things like alfalfa sprouts and bean sprouts but I have grown to love them and to add them to my juices or salads whenever I can. They are really easy to sprout at home; you just need a sprouting jar and some seeds. You can also find them, and other seeds and beans, ready sprouted from most health stores.

Choose organic wherever possible

If your budget allows for it, the organic route is the least toxic and, as fat cells love toxins, you need to eliminate as many outside chemicals and pesticides as you can. Especially if you are juicing vegetables or blending fruit. When you juice, you are not only extracting 90 per cent of the vitamins and minerals but also 90 per cent of any chemicals the vegetable may contain.

On the other hand, I see no point in buying organic kiwi fruit if it's been flown thousands of miles to get to the supermarket shelf, as there won't be many fresh nutrients left.

Use your own common sense, and buy organic wherever possible, but especially vegetables for juicing, and make sure you wash, top and tail and peel anything else that is *not* organic.

Sweat those toxins out

As you may have read earlier, muscles burn calories all the time, even when we're lying on a sofa during a detox weekend! So the more muscle you have, the faster your metabolism will be and the more you will lose weight.

During the Kickstart Detox, exercise is also essential to get rid of toxicity. As the skin is the largest elimination organ in the body, you need to sweat for at least 20 minutes each day of the weekend to throw those toxins out.

Don't forget that exercise also makes you happy because the body releases 'feelgood' hormones called endorphins after 20 minutes of working out – and brisk walking will do the job just as well.

Boost your metabolic rate

As you've seen, exercise will boost your metabolic rate. If you don't exercise regularly, your metabolic rate drops by 2–5 per cent every ten years. So it's important to get into the exercise habit this weekend if you want permanent weight loss.

You will also be boosting your metabolic rate by incorporating essential fatty acids (EFAs) into your daily regime. EFAs increase your metabolic rate and energy levels, helping you to burn more calories, even at rest. Your body goes far further on healthy fats than it does on carbohydrates.

Clean your 'guttering'

The lymphatic system is like the guttering in your body, where all the debris gathers, before being broken down and eliminated. It is a secondary circulatory system running alongside the blood. But unlike the blood, it has no pump of its own so relies on a bit of help to get it moving.

Exercise is one of the best ways to move your lymph, and another is skin-brushing. Your skin, as an eliminating organ, can get rid of more than half a kilo of waste and toxins every day, so get into skin-brushing and get your internal guttering clean over the next 48 hours. You'll learn how to skin-brush a little later in this chapter.

Eat the right amount, at the right time

Two cupped hands full of food equals three quarters of your stomach size, which is the maximum amount your stomach can process at any one time. Please try and stop eating before you're full, when you feel you could eat just a little more, because the signal from the stomach to the brain saying 'I'm full' takes a good 5 minutes. So wait for five and you may well feel fuller than you thought.

Try not to eat again for another 4 hours, so that the last food is properly broken down and secreted into the small intestine. If you eat again within an hour or two after a meal, the body has to leave the previously eaten food half-digested and go and sort out the new arrivals. The previous food starts to ferment and putrefy and hey presto, you've got bloating! The new food is also half-digested, which increases toxicity.

It's a waste of energy, energy that you need to shift those stubborn pints of water!

Switch the outside world off

Take time out from the stresses and strains of the outside world by turning it off, so you can concentrate on detoxing safely and effectively. Switch all your connections with the outside world off for as long as you can bear, so you can really relax while you're cleansing.

If you turn off the phones and the telly for longer than normal, you'll discover extra scope to do all sorts of things for yourself you haven't had time to do before, such as self-massage, acupressure, or just soaking in a warm, scented bath.

It is especially important to turn the TV and phones off around mealtimes, because stress and external stimuli will affect your digestion and you won't be chewing your drinks or drinking your food properly if you are distracted!

But if the weather's lousy and you're really tired, by all means just slump on the sofa with a light movie and snooze away! You may well feel more tired than normal so sleep as much as you like.

TV

Watching TV for several hours excites the nervous system. This in turn can dehydrate you, which can cause your body to hang on to water – bloating. So just have the TV on in the evening for a couple of hours, if it's not warm enough to go for a walk. The less often you have the TV on, the more likely you are to be up and about doing something and burning those calories.

Telephone & laptop

Answering the phone and checking your e-mails may well stress you if you are trying to unwind and concentrate, possibly for the first time in your life, on YOU. So turn both the landline and mobile on to answerphone for those times of the day when you really need to be quiet. If you can pretend to be away for the weekend, so much the better – then you will really have time to unwind and un-tox!

Watch

Again, as this is 'me' time; just take your watch off for the weekend. You won't need it, unless you want to time a technique or treatment. See how it feels to just go with the flow, to get up when you like and to go to bed when you like and sleep when you like. This is supposed to be a home-from-home health spa WITHOUT rushing from one treatment to the next, so go without Father Time for 2 days.

Knickers and bras

The reason I've added this one is because I want you to be as comfortable as possible and to do without tight, restrictive clothing that may be contributing to your fluid retention, especially if it's hot. You don't need elastic digging into you while you relax with a diuretic natural juice in your hands! Go commando and wear comfortable sweats, a sarong, or pyjamas, or nothing at all! It's up to you, it's your weekend. As long as your clothing is loose and cool and comfy enough for you to lounge around and allows you to do some gentle exercise.

Obviously, if you are going out on a strenuous power-walk or trek and you are a woman you will need proper chest support. But while you are indoors, make the most of your 48 hours of freedom.

Let's now look at what you won't need to do during your Kickstart Detox.

On the kickstart detox you will not . . .

Go Hungry
Go Without Protein
Go Without EFAs
Count Calories
Weigh Yourself

Don't go hungry

You won't get hungry on this plan, as long as you make the smoothie in the morning and drink plenty of juices, water and herbal teas in between. If you do get hungry, there are snack suggestions built into your Kickstart Detox weekend: snacks that won't take too much effort for your system to digest.

As explained earlier in the book, fasting and starving play no part in a successful detox. Although I have recommended that you leave at least 4 hours between meals, there is nothing to stop you from filling up with a cup of miso broth or another smoothie in between. Please don't go hungry, but please do try to make your 'filler' a *liquid filler* so your digestion has less to do.

To detox safely and successfully, the liver needs certain amino acids only found in animal protein, so you can have a little protein AND dairy during the weekend.

Don't go without protein

A complete lack of protein in your diet can cause fluid retention because the liver needs the amino acids provided by protein to produce albumin – an essential component for the prevention of water retention.

Protein is also essential for supporting the thyroid, which in turn will support your metabolism.

And although cleansing raw fruits and juices will give you the most rapid water loss, you may also suffer from blood-sugar fluctuations without a little protein at the same time.

If you are a vegetarian, you can replace any of the following proteins with seeds and nuts:

Animal protein – 1 heaped tablespoon a day

Quark – a very low-fat cheese

'Live' yoghurt – you can have cow's, goat's, or sheep's yoghurt.

Cottage cheese – a low-fat cheese

Don't go without EFAs

If you don't have enough essential fatty acids in your diet, your body is more likely to retain excess fluid. In fact, you can't lose weight without Omega 3 and 6 essential fats. They increase metabolism, heat production and energy levels, which means that you burn more calories. Although they are fats, they actually make it harder for your body to *make* fat and easier to *burn* fat.

EFAs help your kidneys to dump excess water held in your tissues – water that appears as extra weight. They also suppress your appetite more than you can imagine as well as preventing carb- and sweet cravings. They'll make you feel happier and lift depression, so you won't *want* to overeat. And they make you feel more like being physically active, so you burn even more calories. Convinced? Good, make sure you have a *minimum* of 2 tablespoons of one of the following oils during your Kickstart Detox. Remember that you CANNOT lose weight without them.

Never, ever heat these oils

Best sources of Omega 3 & 6 essential fats

Flaxseed oil, also known as linseed oil

Flaxseed oil is the richest source of the essential fatty acid most lacking in our diet: Omega 3 (alpha-linolenic acid). It also contains small amounts of the other essential fatty acid we can't make for ourselves: Omega 6 (linoleic acid).

If you're going to use non-fattening oil for your salad dressing, this is the one. You can find a completely *tasteless* flaxseed oil under Resources and a healthy French dressing in the recipe section.

Hempseed oil

Hempseed oil is one of the most balanced oils you can find, as it's high in both Omega 3 and 6.

As it is an acquired taste, I find this oil perfect for adding to a smoothie. Once fruit and lecithin granules are added to your drink, you will not taste the oil at all.

However, if you like the taste of hempseed oil, it's the perfect one to put into your smoothies, drizzle on your food and use in your salad dressing.

Omega 3 & 6 oil blend

Finally, you can also buy a ready-blended Omega 3 & 6 oil that ensures a perfect balance of essential fats. If you find one you like the taste of, you can use it throughout the weekend.

There is more information on oils in chapter 15 and recommended blends under Resources.

Lecithin granules

Lecithin is made from soybeans and works like washing-up liquid, emulsifying the oils. As it is 57 per cent Omega 6 to 7 per cent Omega 3, this is the perfect partner for flaxseed oil. If you have only bought one oil and it's flaxseed, taking lecithin at the same time will ensure you are obtaining the correct balance of Omega 3 and 6 essential fatty acids.

It will also turn your smoothie into a real milk shake, without the milk. So whatever oil you decide to use during your Kickstart Detox, I recommend you add 2–3 heaped teaspoons of lecithin to your smoothie. It's such a good 'food' that your liver and brain should thank you for it, but listen to your body and see how you feel. If you feel nauseous, leave it out. Lecithin granules can be found in any reputable health store.

Other sources of protein & EFAs

Nuts and seeds are also very rich sources of protein and EFAs. These can be eaten regularly, but not in great quantities (unless you are a vegetarian). You can have any UNSALTED nuts and seeds from the list except for peanuts.

Seeds and nuts provide a complete protein for sprinkling on your yoghurt, salads or fruit salad.

! TOP TIP

If seeds are soaked overnight they become more digestible, release their valuable essential fats into the water and become more alkaline.

Also, if you put your nuts and seeds in a wok – without adding salt, oil, water or anything else – and toast them lightly till they pop, they taste crunchier and last longer.

Don't count calories or weigh yourself

The liver holds the key to weight loss and a balanced metabolism. It is the major fat-burning organ in the body and when you detox you are kickstarting it to do its job properly so water and toxicity loss begins naturally and easily.

If you look after your liver by giving it the supporting nutrients it needs, which you will during this detox, there is absolutely no need to count calories, weigh food or even weigh yourself. This whole weekend is about banishing the bloat, not losing fat. Although you probably will lose a couple of pounds or more of water, your clothes will tell you more about the success of your kickstart Detox than your scales will.

The shopping list

So are you ready to shop till you drop? Don't buy anything that is NOT on this list, it's only 48 hours and you *can* live without whatever you're already missing! Apart from your one cup of organic tea or coffee, if you must, the rest of your cravings will go if you have taken your time to get to this point and make sure you follow all the preceding suggestions.

These are the very BEST foods for flushing fluid and toxins out of your body. You obviously don't need to buy all of them, just pick your very favourite fruit and veg so you can stick to this Kickstart Detox.

You'll need at least 6 meals, which can be made up of smoothies, juices, salads or soups. Have a look at the recipes at the end of this chapter, as well as the 'pampering' section, before making your own shopping list.

As an example, I will provide you with my own shopping list later, so you have a clearer idea of the amounts you will need for a weekend. But this is only a guide and very much represents my own taste rather than yours. This is your weekend, so pick only those foods that work for you.

The kickstart shopping list

Food flushers

- Fennel
- Artichoke
- Dandelion
- Dill
- Carrots
- Celery
- Cucumber
- Parsley
- Beetroot
- Nettles
- Lettuce
- Cabbage, Broccoli, Brussels Sprouts, Kale & Cauliflower
- Red Cabbage
- Tomatoes
- Asparagus
- Avocado

- Radishes
- Spinach
- Watercress
- Red, Yellow & Orange
  Peppers

- Chicory
- Alfalfa Sprouts etc
- Leeks

There is one thing I need to mention about fruit. Although fruit is wonderful for detoxing, in some people, such as those suffering from cystitis, Candida or fluctuating blood-sugar levels, fruit can exacerbate the problem. So please listen to your body and if your symptoms worsen or you suffer from bloating, go easy on the fruit and try and incorporate vegetables as much as possible.

If you're making the Smoothie, you can always add 50–100 ml of water to any fruit juice you're drinking, so it is less sugary.

Fruit food flushers

- Watermelon
- Strawberries
- Pineapple
- Apples
- Other Berries
- Black Cherries
- Citrus Pith
- Blackcurrants
- Dark Grapes
- Peaches & Nectarines

- Papaya & Mango
- Pink Grapefruit
- Apricots
- Figs
- Oranges & Tangerines
- Lemon
- Lime
- Kiwi

Supplements & essential fatty acids

Colon cleanser – buy one that includes psyllium husks, pre-biotics and probiotics.

Milk thistle – helps the liver detox safely, see chapter 12 on supplements.

Flaxseed oil, also known as linseed oil – available in some major supermarkets and most health stores.

Or hempseed oil – available in some major supermarkets and most health stores.
Or Omega 3 & 6 blended oil – available in health stores.
Lecithin granules – available in health stores.

Unsalted nuts

Almonds, brazils, cashews, pecans, walnuts, macadamia – any (but not peanuts)

Seeds

Pumpkin, flax, sesame, sunflower seeds and pine nuts. You can buy tubs of these, already mixed and roasted, in most health stores.

Protein

'Live' yoghurt – cow's, sheep's or goat's.
Or quark
Or cottage cheese

Flavourings

Sea vegetables: Dulse, Arame, Wakami or Nori, from health stores
Fresh garlic
Fresh ginger
Turmeric
Mother Hemp pesto: a delicious topping made from hempseed oil & pine nuts or sun-dried tomatoes (Sainsbury's)
Tahini: made from sesame seeds, good for toppings, buy a runny one.

Pampering shopping & other optionals

Essential oils – see suggestions
Epsom bath salts
Natural bristle brush for skin-brushing
Sprouting jar

Drinks

At least 4 litres of mineral water – Volvic and Spa are the lowest in sodium. (Home-filtered water is fine.)
Herbal tea – lemon and ginger is a great liver supporter
Detox tea – make sure it contains liquorice, ginger, dandelion, fennel seeds, or parsley.
Miso instant soup – look for one containing spirulina for more detoxing benefits.

Example of my last shopping list for a 2-day detox

6 lemons	2 pink grapefruit or
6 small beetroot	1 mango & 1 papaya
big chunk of ginger	fresh apricots
2 × 750 g bags of carrots	fresh figs
1 bulb fresh fennel	4 kiwi fruit
75 g bag of watercress	small tin of lecithin granules
parsley – bunch	250 ml flaxseed oil
180 g bag of radishes	250 ml hempseed oil
2 bunches of celery	lemon & ginger herbal tea
2 × 200 g of mixed salad	nettle tea
200 g of rocket	mixed nuts & seeds
large cucumber	garlic
small bag of alfalfa sprouts	6 × 1.5 l bottles of Volvic
(I sprout my own now)	mineral water
4 small avocados	jar of tahini (sesame seed
2 × 250 g tubs of quark	paste)

1 × 500 g tub of 'live'
  yoghurt
2 cartons of organic apple
  juice
750 g bag of apples
punnet of strawberries
punnet of raspberries
1 kg of dark cherries

Nature et Progrès natural
  seasalt
6 × 21 g packets of miso
  spirulina organic instant
  soup
160 g jar of Mother Hemp
  red pesto

(I have Epsom salts, a natural-bristle skin brush, olive oil, sea
vegetables and essential oils etc in stock!)

So you've arrived at the start of your 48-Hour Kickstart Detox.
Hopefully, by now, you will have read through the rest of the
chapter, chosen your recipes, bought your provisions, cut down on a
lot of the external and internal toxins and are ready for a thoroughly
relaxing weekend.

I've outlined an Optimum Plan, to give you an idea about what
to do and when to do it. But it is only a guide and, as I've said
dozens of times, this is YOUR weekend, not mine, so please go
ahead and do exactly what you like and in any order you like. I've
included all the techniques I would use for a Kickstart Weight-Loss
Detox, but do feel free to refer back to previous chapters and go for
an alternative if you prefer.

You don't have to start on a Saturday morning through to Sunday
night. You can take your 48 Hours from any part of the week – as
long as you do it before embarking on any of the 3 weight-loss
plans following this chapter.

Suzi's optimum plan

Wake up naturally
Affirmation
Liver cleanse – hot water and lemon
Washing and tongue-scraping

Liver flush juice

5 Rites Exercises

Skin-brushing & Shower

Cellulite massage

BREAKFAST – Eliminator smoothie

Brisk walking – exercise outside

LUNCH

Post-lunch rest

Afternoon relaxation: reading, walking, and chilling

Yoga exercise for posture

Breathe your Abs flat

Afternoon snack

DRINK WATER THROUGHOUT THE DAY

Facial acupressure

Diuretic Tea

SUPPER

Evening relaxation:

Visualization exercise for cellulite

Bath before bedtime

Spine relaxer

Anti-bloating nightcap

EARLY TO BED

Bedtime visualization

And simply repeat for day two – but feel free to adapt the plan. Do exactly what you want to do, when you want to do it, in any order you like! It's *your* weekend.

Wake up naturally on Saturday morning

Waking up between 5 a.m. and 7.00 a.m. is the best time during a detox because the large intestine 'time', according to Chinese medicine, is between those hours. When you think about it, it makes sense because any toxic waste will have accumulated in the rectum and bladder during the night and will be waiting to come out sometime between 5 a.m. and 7 a.m. or – at worst – between

6 a.m. and 8 a.m. Otherwise, that waste may stay in your gut and be reabsorbed back into the bloodstream.

However, unless it's the height of summer and you wake up naturally at this time, please go ahead and get up when you like. A detoxing body needs lots of rest, so just go with the flow.

Affirmation

This can be done in bed before you get up.

Just say to yourself:

> *I am strong and healthy.*
> *I am opening my eyes to a brand-new day.*
> *I am wide-awake.*
> *I no longer crave sugar (or any other substitute).*
> *I am losing water and toxicity by eating healthy food.*
> *This weekend is the start of my permanent weight loss.*

1st Liver cleanse

Kickstart your liver cleanse by adding the juice of a fresh lemon to 1–2 glasses of hot water. Although acidic, lemon (or lime) juice makes your system *alkaline*, which will help your digestion and get rid of any bloating. Hot water and lemon also stimulates your kidneys, which will start fluid elimination.

Wash

Splash your face with cool/cold water a few times. Vigorously rub a flannel over your face to get rid of any dead cells and toxicity left on your skin overnight.

Tongue-scraping and teeth cleaning

By having a quick look at your tongue every morning, before you clean your teeth, you will be able to see how your digestion is doing.

If you also get into a daily habit of *scraping* your tongue you will be sending a message to your gastric juices and digestion to wake up. As soon as the millions of taste buds on your tongue are stimulated they send a message to the digestive system to get ready and your food will be broken down more efficiently.

To scrape the tongue, use a tongue scraper (sold in health shops or by mail order) or a small spoon or even your toothbrush. Gently scrape from the back of the tongue forward until you have scraped the whole surface. The whole process only takes twenty seconds and will get rid of that unpleasant coating, clear bacteria out of your mouth and make your breath smell sweeter!

Liver flush juice

This should be drunk before you do your Tibetan 5 Rites and within 20 minutes of drinking your glass of hot water and lemon.

If you have a juicer, make one up now from the suggestions in the recipe section. This should be drunk immediately so you obtain all the nutrients that have been extracted from those healthful vegetables.

If you don't have a juicer, you can buy one of the many ready-made vegetable juices instead. Although a lot of the nutrients will have dissipated, juices such as carrot juice will still help support the liver in its detoxification process and you can always add a couple of the suggestions in the recipe section to give it an extra kick.

But if you can, do try and buy a juicer – there are some very reasonably priced ones on sale in supermarkets and in the high street.

Evacuation

Hopefully, you will have done a perfect poo by 7 or 8 a.m. If you haven't, just try this simple yoga exercise that places gentle pressure on the large intestine, which will help to get it going so it will expel the last digested meal.

Bowel mover

Lie on the floor and draw your right knee up to your chest as far as you can, clasping your hands around your knee firmly, with your fingers interlaced. Breathe in deeply and pull your knee, again, gently downwards towards your chest. Breathe out and release your knee, but don't let go. Repeat several times, pulling your knee further into your chest each time you breathe in. Then lower your right leg to the floor. Now repeat the sequence on your left side. Finally, pull both your knees up together and repeat the same sequence several times. Deep breathing is essential.

This should clear any constipation quickly and naturally. But don't worry if you don't go on the first day – the fibre in the colon cleanser, which you are going to add to your breakfast smoothie, should take care of cleaning your internal house for you.

5 Rites exercises

For those of you who are yogis and don't want to get into the Tibetan 5 Rites, you can do six rounds of sun salutations instead. That should get everything moving.

Fellow nutritionist Nor Power taught me the Tibetan 5 Rites. Nor discovered these 5 simple exercises 6 years ago having come across them in a book. She used to do 50–100 sit-ups a day for her abs and other toning exercises for the rest of her body. But, having given the 5 Rites a whirl, she noticed, even after the very first day, that her muscles ached more than they had after her other regime. She had better ab definition just doing 21 of each of the 5 rites than with her previous 100 sit-ups. She felt more energetic and noticed that these simple exercises gave her back, tummy, thighs, arms and shoulders a thorough but quick workout.

The Tibetan monks who originated these exercises many hundreds of years ago believe that an energy centre or vortex covers each of the major 7 glands. Hindus and yogis call them chakras. In a healthy body, each vortex revolves at great speed, allowing life energy, or 'prana', to flow upward through the endocrine system.

But if one of them slows down, the flow of health and vitality gets blocked and that particular gland may not work as efficiently as it should. When they are all revolving at the same speed your nerves, organs and glands will work better and you will have more energy – energy you need if you are to detox successfully and continue to lose weight.

Endocrine glands/chakras

1. The reproductive glands
2. The pancreas
3. The adrenals
4. The thymus
5. The thyroid – metabolism!
6. The pineal
7. The pituitary

These simple 'rites' will wake up your whole endocrine system and, as you are working your whole body using your own limbs as weights, will also tone and strengthen the major muscle groups, serving as a quick muscle-resistant exercise you can do at home.

For the best results they need to be done daily. They will only take 10 minutes to do, once you've learned how to do them this weekend, and within a month of daily practice you should look and feel much better.

Each exercise should be repeated no more than 21 times. But most of us need time to work up to that number so start off with as many as you feel comfortable with and increase the number each week. If you can only manage 3 repetitions over the weekend, that's fine. Increase it to 5 or 6 the following week, and so on.

Always do only what you can handle. Everyone is different, so if you get stuck on nine repetitions and can't seem to get past that number, don't push yourself. Listen to your body and do what you're comfortable doing. It doesn't matter *when* you get to the point of being able to do 21 one after another, as long as you're doing them daily. Eventually you'll be doing 21 in just ten minutes before rushing off to work!

See how many you can do over the weekend and then stick to the *same number for each exercise* for the rest of the week.

EXERCISE 1
Tibetan twirling

This exercise will be familiar to you if you have read *48 Hours to a Healthier Life*. It might make you feel like a mad whirling dervish or a child but it will help wake everything up and is a great stress-buster.

How to twirl

Stand up straight with your arms stretched out to the sides with your palms open and facing downward. Spin round clockwise until you become dizzy – usually 5–6 times the first time. Make sure your feet are squarely on the ground throughout, and spin as fast as you can without falling over.

Stand still at the end and take a couple of full, deep breaths.

To help combat dizziness, you could try the trick that dancers and skaters use. Fix your eyes on an object or a mark on the wall in front of you, level with your eyes, and keep your eyes on that point for as long as possible while you are turning. Your head will have to keep up with your body, but turn your head at the last possible moment really quickly so you can stare at the same spot as you come round. But be careful not to hurt your neck by moving it too quickly.

EXERCISE 2

Lie flat on the floor face up, preferably on a thick carpet or rug. Put your arms down along your sides, palms facing down. Inhale deeply and lift both your legs vertically just past a 90-degree angle, and raise your head off the floor with your chin tucked in. Your toes

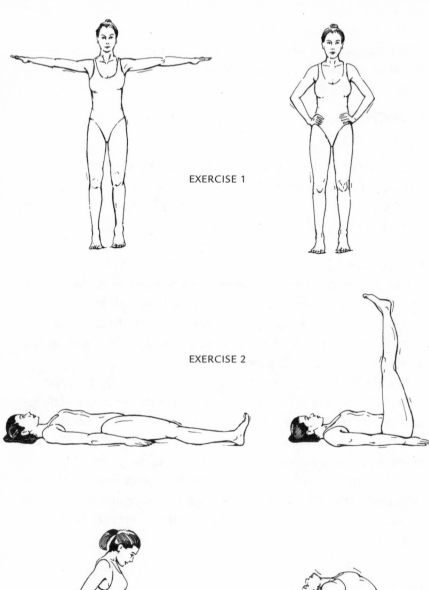

EXERCISE 1

EXERCISE 2

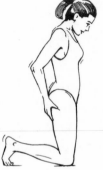

EXERCISE 3

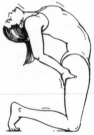

EXERCISE 4

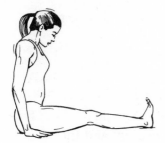

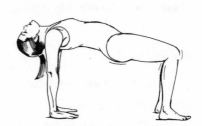

EXERCISE 5

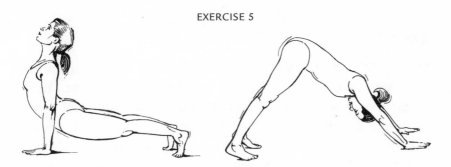

point towards the ceiling and your lower back should remain glued to the floor.

Exhale and lower both your head and legs. Repeat as many times as you can manage. If you can't straighten your knees initially, keep them bent till you can. The important thing is that you are working your abs and thighs, not your neck.

Take two full breaths before moving on to the next exercise.

EXERCISE 3

Kneel on the floor, upright, with your hands on the back of your thighs or just below your bottom. Your knees should be about four inches apart. Look down, tucking your chin in, and then inhale and drop your head as far back as you comfortably can, arching your back from the waist. Your hands will support you as you lean back. Use your arms and hands for support. Exhale as you return to the starting position and repeat as many times as you can.

Take two deep breaths before moving on to the next exercise.

EXERCISE 4

Sit on the floor with your legs straight out in front of you with your feet about 12 inches apart and your back straight. Your palms should be face down on the floor, parallel with your hips. Tuck your chin into your chest. Inhale through the nose, and raise your hips as you bend your knees, raising your whole body up, like a crab. Then drop your head back as far as it will go, tensing your muscles. Your arms should be straight and your feet shouldn't move as you exhale and come down to the starting position. Repeat.

Stand up and take two deep breaths.

EXERCISE 5

The last exercise is the one I find the toughest. It really works the arms, thighs and abs. Lying face down on the floor with arms and legs about 2 feet apart, lift yourself off the floor, as if you are hovering, by supporting yourself on the palms of your hands and the balls of your feet. Your head is up and back.

Inhale and, keeping your arms and legs straight, push yourself up into an inverted V by raising your bottom and tucking your chin into your chest. Exhale as you move back down to the starting position, keeping your body off the ground in that hover position. Repeat.

Stand up and take two deep breaths, then lie down and relax for a couple of minutes till your breath returns to normal.

That's it, five simple exercises that have given your muscles and glands a quick but thorough workout.

Skin-brushing and shower followed by cellulite massage

The skin is our largest organ and, just like the kidneys, liver and colon, it is an *eliminating* organ that can get rid of more than half a kilo (a pound) of waste and toxins each and every day. You don't want the skin choked up and clogged by dead cells during a detox, otherwise toxins stay in the body and the other eliminating organs will have to work harder to clear them.

Skin-brushing is a really simple, quick and effective technique that will give your skin some help eliminating that waste as well as waking up your lymph. It only takes a few minutes and will really Kickstart your Detox this weekend.

Before showering or bathing, on dry skin, start brushing firmly UP TOWARDS THE HEART, starting from the soles of your feet. Work up each leg to your abdomen. Brush your tummy with circular movements in a CLOCKWISE direction. Carry on brushing upwards to the bottom of your chest. Then all the way up the *back* of your legs past your bottom, brushing as vigorously as is comfortable. The bottom and thighs are good areas to concentrate on as, in women, they usually carry the most fat cells!

When you get to your chest and upper back, change the direction and start brushing from the neck DOWNWARDS towards the heart, both front and back. Always in the direction the blood flows towards the heart. Finally, brush your hands and up your arms to the top, front and back, and don't forget to brush *inside* your armpit by holding your arm up and brushing *downwards*.

Don't do your face, but you can give the back of your neck and your scalp a good going-over. You should feel very energized at the end of this technique.

By the end of the weekend, when you can see and feel the benefits of skin-brushing, you will want to find 5 minutes to carry on every morning. Why not start now?

Hot and cold showering

If you haven't invested in a body brush you can always do this technique in the shower to help get the lymph flowing. You can do it as well as skin-brushing, if you like. It will strengthen your immune system and energize you.

Have a shower, and when you have reached the end of your ablutions turn the shower on as cold as you can stand it for 10 seconds (building up to 30 seconds), then turn it up to warm again for a minute or two. Repeat this three or four times and end on cool.

As the hot water warms up your skin, the blood – and therefore the lymph – rushes up to the surface of your body to keep the heat away from precious organs. As the cold water hits the surface of your skin, the blood and the lymph rush *away* from the surface of your skin to protect the organs. So you can see this is a really good way to get things pumping – and it's free!

> 2 minutes warm
> 10–30 seconds cold
> Repeat 3–5 times
> Finish on cool water

After your shower, you can give yourself a quick massage, concentrating in particular on any cellulite areas. The following 'recipe' was put together for you by aromatherapist Vanessa Ough.

Application oil

You will need

- A blending bowl, or wide teacup.
- A vegetable base oil, known as a 'carrier oil': sweet almond oil is probably the most versatile and useful, or grapeseed, safflower, or sunflower. Even a good-quality olive oil will do if you haven't had a chance to buy one of the other oils. For very dry skins a small amount of jojoba, avocado, or sesame oil can be added. Or you can make life even easier for yourself, and buy a 'body milk' which incorporates several nourishing and moisturizing oils. (See Resources.)
- Dark glass bottles, available in various sizes. You can usually get these from a chemist.
- A teaspoon for stirring.
- A plastic measuring cup or jug.
- A sticky label.

'Cellulite' formula – for fluid retention and cellulite reduction

This is a reviving blend, so it is best not to use it past 7 p.m.

Cardamom essential oil	2 drops
Grapefruit essential oil	2 drops
Cypress essential oil	2 drops
Jojoba oil (carrier oil)	5 drops
Carrot oil (carrier oil)	5 drops

Place 30 ml of your carrier oil, such as sweet almond oil, or body milk into a teacup and add 2 drops of each of the above essential oils PLUS 5 drops each of jojoba and carrot oils. Stir the mixture well and pour into a dark glass bottle. Pop a label on so you can continue to use this oil after your Kickstart Detox weekend.

Always work towards the heart, and apply all over your body, as you would a moisturizing lotion, using long sweeping movements.

Pay particular attention to any cellulite areas by kneading the flesh as well as massaging.

Breakfast

Again, according to Chinese organ 'times', in an ideal world a light breakfast should be taken by 9.00 a.m. latest. The best time is between 7 and 9 a.m., which is stomach time. You are quite literally breaking a fast so you need to recharge your batteries and energy levels for the rest of the day. However, you have probably had so much to do during your Kickstart Detox you may well be breakfasting a lot later! Don't worry. As long as it kickstarts your metabolism and raises your blood-sugar levels, it doesn't really matter what time you have breakfast, as long as you don't skip it.

Eliminator smoothie

This is what I make for breakfast every single morning. Because of the ingredients it's a lot more than a simple smoothie: it's so filling that I don't need anything else to eat for at least 5 hours. It also delivers all the vitamins, minerals, fibre, protein and essential fatty acids that your body needs to function and to cleanse.

This is just my version; you can make your own smoothie from any of the recommended fruits and juices (see end of chapter).

Ingredients – place the following in a blender and just whiz up.

> 1 glass of cranberry, prune, apple or apple & mango juice
> Handful of strawberries, blueberries or raspberries
> 2 tablespoons of flaxseed or hempseed oil
> 1 tablespoon of quark, cottage cheese or 'live' yoghurt
> 2 teaspoons of colon cleanser
> 2 capsules of milk thistle (open the capsules and pop the powder straight into the blender)
> 1 teaspoon to 1 dessertspoon of lecithin granules (build up slowly)
> 1 tablespoon of ground seeds: flax, pumpkin, sesame and sunflower

If you don't want a smoothie – and I really hope you do – you can always have an alternative breakfast of fresh fruit salad with a dollop of quark or 'live' yoghurt, and a sprinkling of ground seeds and nuts.

But do make sure you get your daily requirement of the fat-busting Omega 3 & 6 oil by adding it to your salad dressing for lunch or supper.

Exercise

> **WARNING**
> **If you have never exercised regularly before, or have not been active for some time, have a health condition or are seriously overweight, please build up very slowly to 30 minutes a day even if you only start at 5 minutes a day. And please always check with your doctor if you have any doubts.**

If you jog, run or go to a gym regularly then please do carry on with whatever you usually do, provided you have the energy to do it. If you have a bike and want to cycle, go ahead. And if you love dancing, then put on the radio, or a CD, loud and dance away! You choose – it's your time as long as you move your butt for at least 20 minutes, but preferably 30–40 minutes.

For your Kickstart Detox weekend, I am only recommending walking as an exercise because it's safe and easy for anyone to do – and you don't need any special clothes other than walking shoes or trainers.

Walking

Make sure you are wearing really comfortable shoes that you're used to walking in and loose, comfortable clothing, including, if you are a woman, a good bra. Wear layers of clothing so that you can remove something and tie it round your waist if you get hot.

Take anything else you may need such as water and a Pac-a-mac and use a light backpack to carry them. You might also want to take weights with you to turn your exercise into more of a muscle-resistant workout. A bottle of water in each hand will do if you haven't got weights.

If you're not used to walking, just go out and walk a little faster than normal, swinging your arms as you go. Aim to walk as fast as you would to catch a bus. But don't push yourself. Even if you only stride out for 10 minutes and then amble slowly back for another 10 minutes, you will still have got your heart rate up and, hopefully, got those toxins moving.

If you're fit, you need to walk as fast and as far as you can to burn fat and sweat out those toxins. You need to walk fast enough to break out in a gentle sweat but not so fast that you can't carry on a conversation. Pump your arms as you go, preferably carrying weights in each hand so you work your upper body as well as your lower body. Try and walk for 30–40 minutes. And don't forget, the faster you walk, the more energy you use and the more calories you burn. Walking fast will actually burn the same amount of calories as running, without placing as much stress on your joints.

Please cool down and stretch your muscles at the end of your walk.

❗ TOP TIPS FOR WALKING DURING THE
● WEEKEND PLAN

Do your Tibetan exercises first, this will warm up your muscles.
Make sure your head and shoulders are relaxed.
Wear loose comfortable clothes and good trainers or shoes.
Take a Pac-a-mac instead of an umbrella.
Swing your arms to get your heart pumping even more.
Towards the end of your walk, slow down and cool down.
Stretch all the muscles you've been using.

Lunch

For maximum fat-burning you should try and eat within an hour of exercising but not less than 45 minutes after finishing your walk.

Lunch should be eaten between 1 and 3 p.m., which is small intestine time, according to Chinese medicine. The secretion of bile and digestive juices are at their highest at this time so you will absorb the nutrients from your food better and place less of a burden on your digestion.

However, many practitioners believe you should eat nearer to 12 noon and, if you have been up since the crack of dawn, you may well need your main meal of the day much earlier. If you feel like eating at noon and going for a walk afterwards, do it. It's your weekend.

This should be your biggest meal of the day, as your energy peaks now and you are more likely to work it off during the rest of the day. If you take a look in the recipe section, there is a salad I always have for lunch, during a detox, that is composed of as many of the natural diuretic and detoxing vegetables from the list as possible. It's filling and nutritious and will keep you going.

But, again, do your own thing and eat whatever you fancy, as long as it's in the recipe section or taken from the Food Flushers list.

! TOP TIP

If you think you may have a poor digestion, you can help prepare your stomach for its first meal of the day by drinking a small glass of water with one teaspoon of organic, cider vinegar, just before eating. You can also repeat this before supper.

After lunch – rest for 15 minutes

Lie down for at least 15 minutes to give your body a chance to digest that big bowl of greens! To relax properly, simply place your left hand on your abdomen with your right resting lightly on top of it. Just lie in that position for as long as you like. There's no hurry! The longer you give your food to digest, the more energy will be available for you to detox and lose weight.

According to our circadian rhythms – our natural body clock – we have two in-built rhythms of sleep: between **10.00 p.m. and midnight** and between **1.30 and 2.00 in the afternoon**, so if you want to have a little nap now – go ahead. All these years we've been fighting the urge to have a siesta and blaming sleepiness on what we ate for lunch when in fact it was just our circadian rhythms!

Afternoon relaxation

This is your time to do whatever you fancy doing. You can just chill and listen to music. You can read, meditate if you want to, go out for another walk or just lie on the sofa and watch a light movie.

I have included a couple of exercises you might like to try out this afternoon. But as I've said, this is your time to do exactly what you want to do. So do nothing if that's what you feel like doing.

If the weather's good, though, I do recommend that you try and get out again into the sunlight, even if it's only for a short walk. Contrary to what we're told, sunlight is actually very good for you and your endocrine system. Every gland in your body will benefit from a little natural light every day. Sunlight also produces vitamin D, which is needed by our bones to absorb calcium.

The more daylight you get the more serotonin is produced and the more serotonin is produced, the more melatonin will be released during the night: so you'll sleep better and deeper. If it's the height of summer, obviously avoid sunbathing between 11 a.m. and 3 p.m. But in the winter, these are the best hours to catch some rays to avoid seasonal affective disorder and to produce serotonin. Take your sunglasses off in the winter so the light gets into your cells.

So if you can, go out for another 20 minutes, even if it's just to sit on a park bench with your face in the sun.

The mountain pose

For those of us who spend our lives driving or sitting in front of a computer try this simple exercise this afternoon, recommended by my yoga teacher, Stuart Tranter. It's a good one to do after lolling on the sofa for a couple of hours!

Stand up straight and adjust your weight evenly on both feet, lifting the kneecaps, tucking your tailbone in, and pulling your shoulders right back and down. Breathe in and out deeply through your nose, breathing right up to the collarbone. Imagine a thread lifting your head to heaven. Hold the position, then move your shoulders back and down.

> Lift Neck
> Shoulders Back
> Shoulders Down
> Repeat 1–3

Keep repeating the sequence for 5 minutes. You will feel and look slimmer and more relaxed.

Breathing your abs flat!

This is another exercise to try out during the afternoon, which is just great for getting toxins out of your lungs and working the abdominals.

It is a breathing exercise called Khapalbhati (Sanskrit name) that another yoga teacher, Ali Campbell-Hill, taught me.

It will give you energy and wake you up either at the end of the day, if you've been resting, or first thing in the morning to energize you.

Khapalbhati

Sit cross-legged, or on your heels, whichever is more comfortable, and relax your belly with your hands on your knees, your shoulders back and spine straight. Blow out through the mouth as you draw your abs in; imagine you're blowing out a candle that won't go out.

Don't think about inhaling. Just keep blowing that candle out, pulling in the abs each time, very quickly, one after another. Do one set of 30, followed by another set, slightly faster.

Feel the burn?

Afternoon snack

The best snack to have in the afternoon would be another vegetable juice. You should be aiming to have two a day – up to a litre of juice a day. This will really help your liver detox, give you a quick boost of nutrients, and energize you. You can make up your own juice using any combination and amount you like, from the Food Flushers list. You'll find suggestions in the recipe section.

If you really don't fancy a juice as an afternoon snack or don't have a juicer, you can have a snack from the list below. But don't forget the 4-hour rule – it's best not to *eat* for at least four hours after your last meal.

A juice is fine because it goes straight into the bloodstream and needs very little in the way of digesting. But I don't want you to go hungry during this detox, so if you really are starving, have one of the permitted snacks from the list.

Snack list

Cup of miso broth
A small handful of mixed nuts
Half an avocado
A bowl of soup
A couple of figs or apricots with a handful of mixed seeds
A small handful of mixed seeds
One piece of fruit from the list
Raw carrots, cucumber and celery sticks with a little tahini

Personal pampering in your own home spa

Make up your preferred blend of essential oils for your facial acupressure exercise. Choose *three* of the essential oils from this list and blend 2 drops of each, as you did for your morning post-shower massage into 30 ml of your carrier oil or body milk. You don't need a lot of oil, but it will help your fingers to move over your face more easily.

These essential oils are the best for water retention

Juniperberry	Lemon
Cypress	Rosemary
Cedarwood	Spike Lavender
Grapefruit	Cardamom

Acupressure

> **WARNING**
> Don't do this exercise if you are on prescription drugs, pregnant, or ill. Don't apply pressure to any facial cuts or bruises, and if you feel dizzy or unwell whilst doing them, please stop and reduce both the pressure and the time on each point.

Acupressure will stimulate blood circulation and your lymph, making your face look brighter and healthier. It is one of the simplest techniques to help you lose any water retention and tension you may be holding around your face, as well as stimulating your major internal organs, via acupoints on your face, to encourage them to function better. All you need is your hands, a mirror, your preferred blend of essential oils and the diagram in this book.

There are 32 acupressure points on your face and, along with the water, juices, exercise and sleep, you should soon see a difference.

You should be glowing with health and, more importantly, urinating more than normal as you lose fluid retention.

Acupressure points

For each acupressure point, you need to press quite hard, using your fingertip or thumb, leaving the pressure there for a minimum of 20 seconds. Don't forget to do both sides of the face and if there are points on both the left and right – pulsate them at the same time.

After the weekend

Once you have learned this technique, you can easily incorporate it into your normal, busy life, by simply tapping quickly, ten times, on each point as you moisturize your skin in the morning. That should only take 5 minutes and will really help boost a sluggish circulation and get rid of any puffiness you might have.

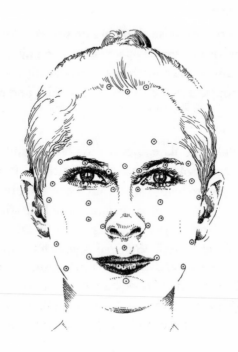

- There are three points right at the top of the forehead. One is right in the centre and the other two are each an inch either side. Press firmly on each point for at least 20 seconds.
- The next point is an inch above the middle of the eyebrow. One each side.
- The next is right in the middle of the eyebrows. Single.
- There is a point right at the end of the outside of the eyebrow. One each side.
- Work inwards, *under* the eyebrow (each side), and press 3 more points – one in the middle, one at the corner just under the beginning of your eyebrow, and the third is right in the corner of your eye, underneath.
- Another one is at the side of the eye, just outside the eye socket. One each side.
- There is one an inch below the middle of the pupil. One each side.
- Another an inch below that. One each side.
- A point either side of the bottom of the nostril. One each side.
- One right above your lip, right in the middle. Single.
- One either side of the outside of your lips, in each corner. One each side.
- One right underneath the middle of your bottom lip. Single.
- One on the side of the face, parallel with the last point. One each side.
- Another point is found on the side of the face just below the ear. One each side.
- And the last one is found on the side of the face, towards the middle of the ear. One each side.

Drink up

Apart from drinking your 2 litres of water a day, afternoon is the best time to drink a natural diuretic tea, such as nettle or dandelion. According to Chinese medicine, between 3 p.m. and 7 p.m. is bladder and kidney time, so you need to drink as much liquid as you can between these times to help flush your kidneys.

You can, alternatively, take 3 dessertspoons of nettle juice, which is available from most health food stores.

Supper and post-supper rest

For maximum weight loss, your last meal of the day should be between 5 p.m. and 7 p.m., the earlier the better, so that you don't go to bed within four hours of eating. That way your digestion will have done its work and your major organs, especially the liver, can spend the night removing toxicity and repairing themselves.

The ideal time to eat supper is 6.00 p.m. because bile secretion and digestive enzymes are drastically reduced *after* this time, causing your digestion to work that much harder.

The less the body has to digest, the more energy it has to cleanse and move toxicity – and therefore fat – out of your cells!

I usually have my smoothie at 8.00 a.m. and my lunch by 2.00 p.m. so by 6–7 p.m. I'm not that hungry and am happy with a big juice. If I get hungry later in the evening, I have a piece of fruit and a handful of seeds and a cup of miso broth to fill me up.

Again, have whatever you fancy. You may want another smoothie, another salad, or soup from the recipe section. It's entirely up to you. Eat exactly what you want, and don't go hungry. There's nothing worse than going to bed on a grumbling tummy!

Evening relaxation techniques

This is your wind-down time. Your chance to practise visualization, affirmations or the lovely half-tortoise exercise that will relax your spine ready for bed. You can also have a delicious aromatherapy bath, in candlelight, or just lie on the sofa and listen to relaxing music. Do whatever you feel like doing. You've always got tomorrow to try out these techniques.

Visualization exercise – a great one for cellulite

This is an exercise I learned at the Bristol Cancer Help Centre whilst on a course in Psycho Neuro Immunology – the link between mind and body. It is a visualization technique for tumours and sickness but I don't see any reason why it wouldn't work as effectively on fat cells and cellulite.

Tune in to the body and feel as if you are in a little boat going wherever you like. Go to where it feels right, not necessarily where there is a physical symptom. Choose a symbol for that part of the body. What does it feel like? Is your cellulite like an animal, fire, sludge etc? It doesn't matter how bizarre your thoughts are – I thought of a green slimy snake (which apparently is quite common). Now imagine you've got to get rid of it. I chopped mine up into bits and then hosed all the debris away with a fireman's hose! Think big and dramatic and powerful.

If it becomes boring, change it. Have fun with it! Breathe into that area. Think of a colour to nourish the area. Then breathe out into the skin and expand it into a zone of healing colour like a bubble. Do it every day for a month, if you can, and note how you feel and how your cellulite is.

Meditation

If you know how to meditate, you could do that instead of, or as well as, your visualization. It will make you feel happier and calmer so you want to continue losing weight for longer.

A bath before bedtime

You can either have an aromatherapy bath, using the essential oils recommended for water retention that you mixed for your facial in the afternoon. Or you can have a real detoxifier – an Epsom salts bath, which completely relaxes your muscles as well as pulling the toxins out. I know which one I'd go for!

You *can't* follow your bath with the cellulite massage you had after your shower this morning as it's too 'reviving'. But you can choose any of the other formulas below and make up your own blend to use instead of body lotion.

Remember to look at the formulas' effects to see if they are relaxing or stimulating. You don't want to use a stimulating blend in the evening.

Light some candles, put on relaxing music and enjoy!

Formula 1 'fatigue'

For fatigue, water retention and helpful for cellulite.
This formula has a balancing effect.
(Do not use in pregnancy.)

Juniperberry	3 drops
Cypress	2 drops
Cedarwood	1 drop

Formula 2 'cleansing'

Particularly for cleansing, decongesting and detoxing and fluid retention. Helpful against cellulite.
A tonic effect, refreshing and uplifting.

Grapefruit	3 drops
Lemon	2 drops
Cypress	1 drop

Formula 3 'circulation'

Enhances blood circulation and good for fluid retention, cellulite, sluggishness, cold hands and feet.
This blend will help ease away aches and pains.
Balancing to relaxing effect.

Rosemary	2 drops
Cypress	2 drops
Spike lavender	2 drops

As before, add 2 drops of your chosen oils to 30 ml of your carrier oil or body milk, ready to use as a body lotion after your bath.

Aromatherapy baths

Use 6–8 drops of your chosen essential oils. Add to your bath water while the hot water's running as the heat will help release the scent. Your bathroom will smell lovely as you bathe and help you relax even more.

If you have sensitive or dry skin, dilute the oils first in a teaspoon of base oil or milk. As oil is not soluble in water, you will need to swish the water really well to disperse the oils.

Soak in your bath for about 20 minutes. You might want to roll up a small towel to support the back of your neck and place a cool flannel on your forehead. Do not use any shampoo or soap until the very end of this treatment. It helps to cool the water down to tepid for the last five minutes.

Have a glass of water to drink afterwards.

Essential oil bath plus Epsom salts

Pour one cupful of Epsom salts (magnesium sulphate) into the bath. Run the water till your bath is nice and deep. Then add six drops of your chosen formula. Swish the water around to dissolve the oils and the Epsom salts.

Don't be alarmed if you have a slight rash after a bath – you will have sweated out toxins and the rash will soon go.

After your bath, moisturize your skin by using one of the essential oil blends instead of body lotion. Simply apply to your whole body as you would any body lotion, with smooth sweeping strokes towards the heart. Apply to the abdomen in a clockwise direction.

Hopefully, you're now wrapped up in a big, fluffy dressing gown ready for bed. Before you turn in for the night, you might want a nightcap and to do the half tortoise exercise to stretch your spine.

If you are suffering from bloating, which may well be a temporary side effect to your body detoxing, try this drink before you go to bed.

Nightcap

Take a tablespoon of freshly chopped parsley and a teaspoon of ground dill seeds in a glass of hot boiling water. Leave for 10 minutes then strain before drinking. Parsley is a natural diuretic and dill seeds help to get rid of gas.

Half tortoise

This is a real must before bed or when you get up in the morning. It will completely relax and open up your spine, unlocking each disc and getting oxygen and blood into each vertebra.

You may want to do this on a towel. Sit on your knees with your spine very straight. Stretch both hands and arms right up above your head as high as you can with your arms glued to your ears and your palms together. Stretch forward as far as you can go till your arms, hands and forehead touch the ground. Sit there with your eyes closed for a full **5 minutes**, breathing deeply in and out.

Early to bed

The old adage, an hour before midnight is worth two hours after, is good to remember for the duration of your 48-Hour Kickstart Detox. So try and get to bed between 10 p.m. and 11 p.m. as the liver's detoxing time, according to Chinese medicine, is between 1 a.m. and 3 a.m. You want to be well into your REM sleep by 1 a.m. so the liver can get on with detoxing without any of the energy it needs going off to do something else.

And try this lovely visualization, devised by T'ai Chi Ch'uan teacher Penny May, before you go to sleep. Do it after your bath and you'll sleep the sleep of the dead!

Penny's bedtime visualization

This is to wash away the day and leave you ready for a peaceful sleep. Get into bed, lying down flat on your back with your feet uncrossed and your arms by your sides. Imagine a white light flowing all the way through your body, from your feet to your head or your head to your feet. Whichever feels the best. Keep this flowing through the body until you feel relaxed and sleepy. You have cleared away the day!

You've now reached the end of the first day of your 48-Hour Kickstart Detox. All you need to do is go back to the beginning and do it all again on the second day. You can try some of the techniques you didn't get a chance to try before, or just repeat what worked best for you – even if it was just sleeping all day! A detoxing body needs lots of rest, so please don't worry if that's all you've done for the entire weekend.

Once you've reached Sunday night or Monday morning, try on some tight jeans. Hopefully, they will be looser by now and you will look and feel a lot slimmer, brighter, and energized – ready to continue with the detox for longer, or go straight on to one of the other weight-loss plans.

Or maybe you just wanted to lose a bit of bloating for that special event and you can now squeeze into that tight little black number without everything hanging out!

If you have done the 48-Hour Detox as a 'quick fix', make sure to eat very gentle, light food for a couple of days following your cleanse. You will find plenty of vegetarian suggestions in the recipe section of the next chapter, but you can also eat a little chicken or fish with plenty of vegetables and cleansing grains such as rice or quinoa. And don't forget to keep drinking 2 litres of water a day.

Either way, I hope you have enjoyed your Kickstart Detox weekend and are now ready to kickstart the rest of your life, whether it involves more detoxing or further weight loss. All right, go on, weigh yourself, I know you're dying to!

Recipes

Reminders and guidelines for the weekend

> Top and tail all vegetables and fruit, especially if juicing and using non-organic produce
> Don't cook with any of the Omega 3 and 6 oils
> Soak nuts and seeds for 30 minutes
> The only salt to use is unprocessed, natural sea salt
> Tamari can be used as a salt substitute
> Use almonds as a thickener for soups etc
> Use miso instant broth to fill up in between meals

As you know, your Kickstart Detox weekend should be composed of as many of the natural diuretics as possible. At the top of your food pyramid should be raw green vegetables, then other raw vegetables, then fruit, then seeds and nuts in moderation only. For maximum inch loss, I would recommend as many 'liquid' meals as possible, such as vegetable juices, soups and fruit smoothies.

You can eat as many of the suggested vegetables as you need to fill you up, but your secret weapon for any vegetable-based meal is the French dressing, see recipe below. If you use flaxseed or hemp-seed oil you will feel much fuller than you usually do after a salad. Unlike olive oil, you can have as much of these oils as you like as YOU CAN'T LOSE WEIGHT AND FLUID RETENTION WITHOUT THEM.

Here's a reminder of the superfoods you need for a successful Kickstart Detox. Those that are particularly suitable for juicing are marked with a 'J'.

Food flushers

Fennel[J]	Red, Yellow & Orange
Artichoke	Peppers
Dandelion	Lettuce
Dill	Cabbage, Broccoli,
Carrots[J]	Brussels Sprouts, Kale &
Celery[J]	Cauliflower
Cucumber[J]	Red Cabbage[J]
Parsley[J]	Tomatoes
Beetroot[J]	Asparagus
Radishes[J]	Avocado
Spinach	Chicory
Watercress[J]	Alfalfa Sprouts etc[J]
Nettles	Leeks

Fruit food flushers

Watermelon[J]	Papaya & Mango
Strawberries	Pink Grapefruit[J]
Other Berries	Apricots
Pineapple	Figs
Apples[J]	Oranges & Tangerines[J]
Black Cherries	Lemon[J]
Citrus Pith[J]	Lime
Blackcurrants	Kiwi
Dark Grapes	
Peaches & Nectarines[J]	

ELIMINATOR SMOOTHIE

Ingredients – place the following in a blender and just whiz up.

1 glass of apple, prune, cranberry, apple or apple & mango juice
Handful of strawberries, blueberries or raspberries
2 tablespoons of flaxseed or hempseed oil

1 tablespoon of quark, cottage cheese or 'live' yoghurt

2 teaspoons of colon cleanser

2 capsules of milk thistle (open the capsules and pop the powder straight into the blender)

1 teaspoon to 1 dessertspoon of lecithin granules (build up slowly)

1 tablespoon of mixed, ground flax, pumpkin, sesame and sunflower seeds

Recommended juices

If you have a juicer, you can juice most of the vegetables and a lot of the fruits from the list and extract and absorb some **90 per cent of the vitamins and minerals** they contain. **As said, I've marked the vegetables and fruit that are suitable for juicing with a J.** The unmarked vegetables are quite bitter, but can be eaten raw or steamed instead.

If you don't own a juicer, you can always *blend* a selection of the more 'watery' fruits, as below. But try and invest in a juicer because they can be bought quite cheaply and vegetable juice is better for fluid elimination than fruit – especially if you suffer from blood-sugar problems.

JUICE FOR MAXIMUM RELIEF OF WATER RETENTION

2 large carrots

4 stalks of celery

¼ cucumber

Handful of parsley

Handful of watercress

Handful of alfalfa sprouts

1 cored apple

Chunk of fresh fennel

Piece of fresh ginger

¼ lemon, including the pith

Big chunk of red cabbage

LIVER FLUSH – SUGGESTED JUICE

The most important foods to help the liver detox are beetroot, radishes, watercress and ginger, because they help drain the liver by stimulating the gall bladder. If you can brave it, add one dessertspoon of olive oil to this juice because it is very high in phytonutrients, which benefit the liver, gall bladder and digestion.

> 1 small beetroot
> 4 carrots
> 4 sticks of celery
> Handful of fresh watercress
> 6 radishes
> Chunk of ginger
> 1–2 apples to sweeten
>
> **Optional**
> 1 dessertspoon of olive oil
> 2 teaspoons of freshly squeezed lemon juice

If you don't have a juicer

Blend:

> 3 small, cored apples
> 2 slices of pineapple
> 6 strawberries
> Half a pink grapefruit, including the pith
> The flesh of half a melon along with a few of the melon seeds

Salad as a main meal

From the list of vegetables, choose any and as many as you like to make up a big bowl of salad. An avocado is highly recommended as it's very filling, highly nutritious and a 'good' fat. Don't forget it is a 'live' food high in lipase, an enzyme that is key for weight loss.

(Other foods rich in lipase are soaked seeds and nuts and 'live' yoghurt.)

This is my favourite salad. As you can see, I'm mad about grating! For some reason, grated vegetables seem much more filling and interesting than cubes of raw food. Especially when smothered in a French dressing that does *not* put on weight.

SUZI'S SALAD

> 200 g packet of mixed salad leaves: rocket, dandelion, sorrel, watercress, cos, mustard greens etc
> 2 grated carrots
> ½–1 grated beetroot
> ¼ grated red cabbage
> 1 small avocado
> Handful of alfalfa sprouts
> 1 tablespoon quark or cottage cheese

You can add pumpkin seeds, pine nuts, and any other seeds you fancy to fill you up with health!

SUZI'S DRESSING

> 1 teaspoon of olive oil
> 2–3 tablespoons of Omega 3 & 6 oil
> 1 dessertspoon of cider vinegar
> 1 small clove of crushed garlic
> Pinch of natural sea salt – I recommend Nature et Progrès Seasalt – if you must!

I have added a teaspoon of olive oil to make the dressing taste like the real thing – it fools everyone who's ever eaten one of my salads, they have no idea it's healthy oil. Hopefully, you will have experimented before the weekend to see which oil you like the most. Personally, I always use a tasteless, flaxseed oil (see Resources) for this dressing and hempseed oil in my morning smoothie. But the choice is yours.

TAHINI SAUCE & RAW VEGETABLES

> 1 tablespoon of the lightest, runniest tahini paste you can
> find (sesame seeds)
> 2 cloves of crushed, fresh garlic
> Juice of 1–2 lemons
> A little soya milk if needed

Just whiz up in the blender and serve with a plate of your favourite
vegetables from the list, cut into batons.

Soups

I have included soups in this section because you may find the
regime too 'empty' or the weather too cool. Here are just a few
suggestions as alternatives to juices and smoothies.

We've all heard about the Cabbage Soup Diet: 10–15 lb lost in 7
days, eating as much cabbage soup as you can stomach. If you can
stomach it, you can make your own version out of any of the
vegetables from the list as they are all natural diuretics and will fill
you up as well as warming you.

Liquids don't need as much energy to digest, so go ahead and make
a big soup that will keep you going between meals and encourage
your kidneys to eliminate more water, safely. My personal favourites
would be watercress, parsley, cabbage, fennel, dandelion (if you can
find some wild, tender leaves growing near you), and celery.

CLEANSING VEGETABLE SOUP

> 3 cups of vegetable stock
> 3–4 spring onions, finely sliced
> 2 bunches of watercress, chopped
> $\frac{1}{2}$ savoy cabbage, finely sliced
> $\frac{1}{4}$ fennel, finely chopped
> Handful of dandelion leaves, torn
> Bunch of parsley, chopped

> 200 ml 'live' yoghurt or quark
> Tamari or sea salt to taste
> Lemon or lime juice to taste
> Fresh herbs to taste
> 1 tablespoon of sea vegetables
> Garlic, cayenne pepper & ginger to taste

Heat the cup of stock in a large pan. Add the onions and herbs, cover and simmer for 5 minutes. Add all the vegetables to the pan and simmer for 10 minutes. Turn off the heat and add yoghurt or quark. Stir well and leave for 5 minutes. Blend until smooth and creamy. Reheat and add lemon or lime juice and Tamari or a little natural sea salt according to taste.

CLEANSING BROTH

This may seem a bit strange because the soup is mainly made up of vegetable peelings! But it's worth a try as the peelings make it extremely high in potassium, which will help shift excess fluid out of the cells.

> Three cups potato peelings
> Three cups carrot peelings
> Three cups chopped, peeled onions and 2 garlic cloves, finely diced
> Three cups chopped celery and dark greens
> 1 chilli, remove seeds and chop very finely
> 1 cup sea vegetables

Place ingredients in a large pot. Cover with water. Bring to the boil and simmer very slowly for one hour. Strain and drink a cup of the liquid. Refrigerate the rest and heat up whenever you want a cup of cleansing broth!

This soup is a little more filling, but is still cleansing and high in protein and nutrients.

SPINACH AND AVOCADO CHILLED SOUP

(Serves 6 so this will keep you going through the weekend!)

>   85 g bag of spinach, roughly chopped
>   500 ml soya milk
>   500 ml vegetable stock
>   250 ml quark or 'live' yoghurt
>   2 ripe avocados
>   Dash of Tabasco
>   Juice of 2 limes
>   Flat-leafed parsley for garnish
>   Ground almonds or cashews to use as a thickener, if
>   necessary
>   Pinch of natural sea salt to flavour or Tamari
>   Omega 3 oil to drizzle over the soup, once it's taken off the
>   heat

Chop off the spinach stalks, wash leaves and place in pan with a little water. Seal with lid and cook for 5 minutes. Stir once, when it is wilted. Drain well and let it cool. Squeeze out the water and chop up the spinach. Place the spinach and flavouring in a large saucepan, stir and then add the soya milk and stock. Add ground cashews or almonds if the soup needs to be thicker. Bring to the boil, cover and simmer for 10 minutes, stirring occasionally.

Leave to cool, purée and pour into bowl. Peel and stone the avocados and purée them with a little of the soup. Stir this into the rest of the soup. Cover with clingfilm and chill in fridge for 2 hours.

To serve, add Tabasco, Omega 3 oil and lime juice. Stir in quark or 'live' yoghurt for marble effect.

You can make chilled soups out of most of the vegetables on the list: asparagus, celery, beetroot, watercress – they all make wonderful summer soups if you get really bored with juices. As a rough guide:

> 4 cups of your chosen vegetable – cooked and puréed
> 4 cups of vegetable stock
> 1–2 tablespoons of lemon juice
> 1 tablespoon of ground almonds or cashews IF thickener is required
> Pinch of natural sea salt or Tamari
> 1 tablespoon of sea vegetables

Combine all the ingredients and simmer for 5–10 minutes. Leave to cool.

GAZPACHO

This is delicious and cooling in the summer and quite filling.

> 1 small, finely chopped red onion
> 3–4 tomatoes
> 1 red pepper, de-seeded
> 1 cucumber
> 1–2 tablespoons of cider vinegar, to taste
> 1 teaspoon of olive oil
> 3 tablespoons of tasteless flaxseed oil or hempseed oil
> 2 cloves of garlic
> Pinch of natural sea salt
> ½ can tomato juice
> 2 spring onions, finely chopped
> Fresh parsley and basil

Peel and de-seed the tomatoes. Purée or blend the chopped onion, tomatoes, half the red pepper, and half the cucumber. Add vinegar, oil, garlic, tomato juice, and seasoning to taste. Finely chop the spring onions, the rest of the cucumber and red pepper and fresh herbs and add to top of the soup. Refrigerate. Add sunflower or pumpkin seeds to the soup, instead of croutons, if you need some crunch!

TZATZIKI

> 250 g of 'live' yoghurt per person
> Half a cucumber, finely chopped
> 1–2 cloves of garlic
> 1 teaspoon chopped, fresh mint
> Lemon juice to taste
> Pinch of natural sea salt
> Hempseed oil or flaxseed oil to drizzle

Mix all the above ingredients together and drizzle the oil over. Enjoy this as a snack served with crudités or as a side dish with your big salad.

VEGETABLE KEBABS

Cube any, and as many as you like, of your favourite vegetables. Drizzle a tiny amount of olive oil over them and sprinkle with herbs and spices before cooking and just pop on the barbecue. Peppers, fennel, tomatoes, and even broccoli are particularly tasty.

Serve with a big green salad.

14.

Long-Term Detox

If you enjoyed the cleansing effect of the Kickstart Detox Weekend and would like to carry on for longer, this is the plan for you. You obviously can't live on juices and smoothies for longer than a few days, especially in the winter, so you will find plenty of non-animal proteins reintroduced to help you follow this regime for far longer without becoming bored to death with it.

First, here's a reminder of the quiz you answered at the beginning of the book. Do the quiz again to see if your answers have changed much since doing the Kickstart Detox Weekend.

Carry on with the detox

I get up every night to urinate
I don't move my bowels every day
I have aches and pains in my muscles and joints
I crave salty foods such as cheese, crisps and olives
I take painkillers for headaches every week
I have cellulite
I live on fast food and takeaways
I drink alcohol every night
I have IBS symptoms
I often suffer from indigestion

Results

More than 4 yeses – you really need to carry on with the detox (with some welcome additions) for a *maximum* of six weeks. This will give your liver a chance to completely regenerate which, in turn, will help your whole body function better and lose weight more easily. This regime is particularly suited to vegetarians, vegans and readers who like pulses and grains. A longer detox plan will also increase your immunity and give you all the benefits you can expect from a detox, as well as healthy weight loss.

How long

The length of time you decide to follow this detox for is entirely up to you. One day is good, one week is even better. A *minimum* of three weeks and a *maximum* of six weeks are just the best. The longer you do it, the more rubbish and weight you'll lose. But it's harder to follow a detox for weeks on end in the real world because socializing and eating out can be a bit of a challenge. Before you decide what length of detox will fit in with you and your lifestyle, have a look at the benefits of a longer cleanse and the meal suggestions at the end of this chapter. It might be less daunting and more do-able than you think.

Why detox for longer

Detoxing is like 'taking time off work' as it gives the body a chance to rest and cleanse. And, as you know from taking a holiday, the longer you rest – the longer the benefits last. Resting the digestion allows energy that would be used to break down food to be redirected to the cells and tissues so they can repair themselves by cleansing. Cleansing allows the lymph, blood, and organs to clear out old, defective, or diseased cells and unneeded chemicals and toxins. The more you clear out the more weight you'll lose and the better you'll feel. As the new, healthy cells grow, the organs start regenerating and your levels of immunity, vitality, and resistance to illness just soar.

The liver can completely regenerate itself in just 6 weeks, even if it's lost up to 90 per cent of its structure. It can still rebuild itself as a functioning organ given the right foods. So if you can, try and follow the detox plan for the full 6 weeks. Your liver will thank you for it and repay you with successful weight loss and improved health and energy.

A cleansing regime that lasts for 3–6 weeks will still benefit you beyond your expectations. If you bite the bullet for a minimum of three weeks, the detox will purify your blood, clean your organs, improve your metabolism and eliminate years of toxic build-up that has made a home in your fat cells. So do try and stick to as much of the detox plan as possible, for as long as possible, for maximum toxicity- and weight loss.

Don't forget that excess weight is waste: waste in the colon and waste in the fat cells. The longer you can chip away at that waste, the more thoroughly you'll get rid of the weight. But if you can only manage a week or so, that's fine – you'll still reap the benefits and you can always move on to one of the other weight-loss plans afterwards.

Before we look at all the new foods you can now reintroduce, let's just remind ourselves of what *not* to have for a successful detox.

What not to have

> Nicotine & caffeine
> Alcohol
> Sugar
> Processed foods
> Saturated fats
> Salt – that includes crisps!
> Wheat – biccies, pasta, cereal, bread, noodles, couscous
> White rice
> Dairy products – with the exception of 'live' yoghurt, quark
>   or cottage cheese
> Meat, fish & eggs
> Fizzy drinks & squashes

A reminder of why these foods are eliminated

Nicotine and caffeine: both obviously toxins, especially *instant* coffee. Both nicotine and caffeine encourage raging blood-sugar levels and water retention. But if you're *really* missing your daily cup of coffee and can't function at work, make it a once-a-day pick-me-up, preferably ground, real coffee and organic.

Alcohol: is broken down by the liver into acetaldehyde, a toxin that will affect the liver cells and increase free radical production. If you're finding it impossible to go without, you can have the *very occasional* glass of champagne or wine, but don't forget it acts as a diuretic and won't help your detoxification process and weight loss at all.

Sugar: causes fluctuating blood-sugar levels and exhausts our adrenals, making us exhausted, foggy-headed, moody and water-retentive. If you can eliminate all sugar and artificial sweeteners for a couple of weeks, your cravings will go.

Processed food: any processed or ready-made food is going to be loaded with unnatural forms of salt, sugar, saturated fat, additives and preservatives. Avoid anything that you're not sure of while detoxing. Check all labels very carefully, even the ones from the organic section, which can still be loaded with salt, sugar or fat.

Saturated fats: cheese, lard, suet, bacon and fatty meats will go straight on to our thighs and harden our arteries if eaten in excess. They're also hard to digest.

Salt: causes fluid retention and bloating, except for the natural sea salt recommended in the previous chapter, *in moderation*.

Wheat: think how flour mixed with water turns into a spongy, chewing-gum-like material which literally sticks to anything. This is what is going on in your gut, so a very good reason to do without it, whether you're wheat-intolerant or not.

White rice: it may be more digestible than wheat but there is very little nutrition in it because the healthiest part of the grain has been taken away and it's usually been bleached, cleaned, oiled and coated.

Dairy products: are difficult to digest, which can cause bloating and excess mucus. You can incorporate *a little* organic goat's or sheep's cheese if you need to. But for the duration of your detox, they are best avoided as much as possible because they're VERY high in salt. Don't forget, you can still have a little quark, cottage cheese or 'live' yoghurt every day for essential protein.

Meat, fish & eggs: avoid while you are detoxing as they're very hard work for your digestion and are quite acidic. Although oily fish is rich in essential fatty acids, it is an acidic food if eaten to excess and will, over the years, build up mucus in the gut. For the cleanest, slimmest gut cut out meat, fish and eggs for 3–6 weeks.

Fizzy drinks & squashes: unless organic, they are likely to be loaded with unnatural flavourings, colourings and additives. Fizzy drinks also bloat the cells, so avoid wherever possible.

Now for the good news! You can reintroduce a lot of foods that were excluded during the 48-Hour Kickstart Detox: foods that are high in protein and low in 'starchy' carbohydrate, so you will obtain all the nutrients you need without becoming water-retentive and bloated.

First, here's a reminder of the best foods for flushing toxicity and water retention out of your system:

What to eat

Food flushers

Fennel	Red, Yellow & Orange
Artichoke	Peppers
Dandelion	Lettuce
Dill	Cabbage, Broccoli, Brussels
Carrots	Sprouts, Kale &
Celery	Cauliflower

Cucumber	Red Cabbage
Parsley	Tomatoes
Beetroot	Asparagus
Radishes	Avocado
Spinach	Chicory
Watercress	Alfalfa Sprouts etc
Nettles	Leeks

Fruit food flushers

Watermelon	Peaches & Nectarines
Strawberries	Papaya & Mango
Other Berries	Pink Grapefruit
Pineapple	Apricots
Apples	Figs
Black Cherries	Oranges & Tangerines
Citrus Pith	Lemon
Blackcurrants	Lime
Dark Grapes	Kiwi

Supplements & essential fatty acids

Colon cleanser – buy one that includes psyllium husks, pre-biotics and probiotics.

Milk thistle – helps the liver detox safely, see chapter 12 on supplements.

Flaxseed oil, also known as linseed oil – available in some major supermarkets and most health stores.

Or hempseed oil – available in some major supermarkets and most health stores.

Or Omega 3 & 6 blended oil – available in health stores.

Lecithin granules – available in health stores.

Flavourings

Sea vegetables: Dulse, Arame, Wakami or Nori, from health stores
Fresh garlic
Fresh ginger
Turmeric
Onions

Carbohydrates

Grains – brown rice, quinoa, spelt & millet
Rice cakes
Rye crispbreads
Oatcakes
Spelt or rye bread – no more than 2 small slices a day
Rice noodles
Buckwheat

Proteins

Pulses such as chickpeas (hummus) or mixed beans add a healthy protein to your meal. No more than 60 g a day.
Tofu and soya products make a healthy alternative to burgers, sausages and even mayonnaise!
Cottage cheese, quark or 'live' yoghurt – 1 small portion a day.

Unsalted nuts

Almonds, brazils, cashews, pecans, walnuts, macadamia – any (but not peanuts)

Seeds

Pumpkin, flax, sesame, sunflower and pine nuts. You can buy tubs of these, already mixed and roasted, in most health stores.

Fruit

Dried fruit – in moderation only and only *with* food, not on its own
Bananas – once or twice a week

Vegetables

Any vegetables in the recipe section: aubergine, mushroom etc
Root vegetables in moderation
Sweet potato or potato – once or twice a week

Extras

Miso – After a couple of weeks of miso broth taken once or twice daily, the body's elimination processes really kick in to get rid of all the stored wastes from the cells, so carry on drinking a mug a day.
Almond, rice or soya milk
Nut butter
Sauerkraut
Umeboshi plums

When it comes to fruit and vegetables, the same rules apply. Make raw fruit and veg, juices and soups the mainstay of your plan, especially if you are doing a longer detox during the summer. Fruit and vegetables help you to eliminate quicker via the colon and kidneys and are practically no-calorie, no-fat foods, high in water.

If you're doing a longer detox during the winter, you can make your meals more substantial by adding any of the recommended grains, the most cleansing of which is brown rice, which sweeps through your intestines, like a broom, removing waste and toxicity.

Protein foods

You will need more protein, such as tofu, pulses, seeds and nuts, but make sure you have no more than 60 g a day of pulses or nuts as they can be quite acidic and fattening.

Pulses

For vegetarians and for the duration of this plan, legumes or pulses are a very cheap but rich source of protein, carbohydrate and fibre. But they are what is called an 'incomplete' protein because they do not have all eight of the essential amino acids, which make up *complete* proteins. To make them complete proteins, pulses need to be eaten with grains. The best example is baked beans on (wheat-free!) toast. Or hummus and brown rice.

Get ready-cooked, canned pulses to save time and to reduce wind. And don't forget hummus is made from chickpeas, which will make it an easy option when you're looking for a high-protein food at lunchtime.

Chickpeas	Black-eye Beans
Pinto Beans	Lentils
Flageolet Beans	Split Peas
Kidney Beans	Soybeans

Tofu

Tofu is fermented soybean, lower in protein and other nutrients than the soya bean but still with very good levels of calcium, iron and potassium. It is also rich in phytoestrogens, which are natural plant oestrogens that act on the body as antioxidants as well as helping women maintain hormonal balance.

People always think of tofu as that white plasticky stuff, silken tofu, that tastes like . . . nothing! But there is now a growing range of tasty tofu products available in supermarkets and health stores such as sausages, frankfurters, rissoles, burgers and other nutritious snacks which taste nearly as good, if not better, than the real thing. You can even find tofu cheesecake in some health stores, and it's really yummy!

Golden rules

Eat your sprouts!

You have learned about the benefits of alfalfa and other sprouts such as radish and mung bean during your weekend detox, so now is the time to get into growing them yourself at home. (Don't worry if you don't have time, there are plenty of ready-grown ones on sale in health stores.)

They are quick and easy to grow at home and you don't even need a garden, just some seeds, water and air.

Most health stores sell a container, complete with seeds, which does all the work for you. You just rinse the seeds, leave them, repeat over a couple of days and hey presto, they start sprouting. Then you have real 'live', energy-packed food that you can add to salads or juices or both.

Alkaline foods

Eating mostly alkaline foods gives us more energy and it takes energy to lose weight, so try to concentrate on these alkaline foods more than the more acidic foods:

Raw fruits	Sea vegetables
Vegetables	Algae
Sprouts	Lima beans
Raw almonds	Aduki beans
Almond butter	Millet
Miso	

Acidic foods – don't pig out on these!

> All other pulses – become alkaline if soaked
> All other grains – become alkaline if soaked
> All other nuts – become alkaline if soaked
> Soya & tofu products

Eat fermented foods

Fermented foods are very important to help get those active enzymes working so that your food is better digested. As well as your pre-meal salad or vegetable juice, it's a good idea to add: raw sauerkraut (make sure it contains no added sugar), 'live' yoghurt, or umeboshi plums or plum paste. You can add any of these to your salads, sauces, soups or cooked vegetables.

Detoxing in the real world

Breakfast ideas

> A fruit smoothie
> Yofu with fresh berries and seeds
> 'Live' yoghurt with fresh berries and seeds
> Wheat-free muesli with rice milk
> Millet flakes or quinoa with almond milk

Lunch ideas

You will find all these foods in major supermarkets or health stores and many of them in the healthier takeaway chains.

> Stuffed vine leaves
> Vegetable soup with rice cakes
> Hummus with raw vegetable batons
> Tzatziki with raw vegetable batons
> Aubergine salad with raw vegetable batons
> Avocado dip (guacamole) with raw vegetable batons

Falafel with hummus

Small baked potato with avocado or cottage cheese

Wheat-free sandwiches, avocado, hummus and carrot or
salad filling

A mixed bean salad

Vegetarian sushi

Supper ideas

*Try to have a fresh vegetable juice before your meal – it will fill you
up, produce natural digestive enzymes and supply you with rocket
fuel, energy-wise.*

Soya bean burgers with salad and a little potato salad

Tofu sausages stir-fried with mixed vegetables

Tofu frankfurters with potato salad

Roasted vegetables with brown basmati rice

Soup and salad, served with rice cakes or wheat-free bread

Vegetable kebabs

Watercress, spinach, rocket and avocado salad with a
sprinkling of goat's cheese

If you are eating out

This is a tricky one as you cannot get away from animal products
or wheat unless you go to a vegetarian restaurant. Most people are
very accommodating, but make sure you've had a snack or a
vegetable juice at home first, just in case.

Starter

You can usually find a vegetable soup or melon as a starter.

Main course

For the main course, ask for a big plate of salad, with avocado, or
cooked vegetables without the meat, fish or cheese.

Pudding

And for pudding, ask for a mixture of seasonal fruit.

You can munch on olives and unsalted nuts if you're still hungry.

Snacks

> Fresh fruit – 1 piece only (bananas only 2–3 times a week)
>
> Crudités: carrot, celery, cucumber or any from the vegetable list, with hummus or tzatziki
>
> Rice cakes, rye crispbreads or oatcakes with hummus, tomatoes, avocado, tahini, vegetarian pesto
>
> A small handful of nuts – NOT salted and NOT peanuts
>
> A small handful of seeds
>
> A few olives
>
> Raisins or sultanas, or dried fruit – STRICTLY IN MODERATION
>
> Soaked prunes or apricots

Drinks

> Lemon and hot water
>
> Fruit smoothie
>
> Vegetable juice
>
> Mug of miso broth
>
> Herbal teas
>
> Green tea
>
> 2 litres of room-temperature water a day

Finally, try and continue the techniques you learned during your 48-Hour Kickstart Detox for maximum detoxification, weight loss and a stress-free life.

AND DON'T FORGET TO DO YOUR:

Tibetan 5 rites – these are muscle-toning and energizing exercises, so try and continue them each day. It will only take you 5 minutes and will set you up mentally and physically for the day.

Skin-brushing – every day before your shower this will clear away any toxicity and dead cells gathered on your skin overnight.

2 litres of water a day – will keep flushing toxicity out of your body and give you lovely clear skin and sparkling eyes!

Liver flush or smoothie daily – or both – will give your body all it needs to continue detoxing safely.

Four hours of exercise a week – essential if you really want to burn fat as well as detoxing successfully. Remember that you need to sweat to get toxicity out of your body.

Sauna – will also get you sweating, so consider having one of these to help your detox on its way. But this is NOT a replacement for exercise!

Your favourite relaxation technique from the weekend – choose an exercise you particularly liked during the Kickstart Detox and practise it daily.

Colonic – do consider having a colonic at the end of your detox. It will help clear your colon of any toxicity that has gathered there and is the best treat you can give your gut after a cleanse!

If you incorporate as many of the above as you can, on a regular basis, your detoxification will go far deeper and clear more 'waste' (and therefore weight) than if you don't do anything else. The more effort you put into this programme, the more weight you'll lose, it's as simple as that!

Once you've finished your 3–6 week detox and everyone's commenting on your glowing skin and shiny eyes and new trim figure, you may well find that you want to carry out a similar detox a couple of times a year. Or you may find that you would like to do a mini-cleanse once a week, or a weekend once a month. Whatever you decide to do in the future, you now know how much of an effect toxicity has on your weight, so here are some tips on how to accomplish mini-detoxes on a regular basis. Good luck!

How to do a quick detox in the real world

Aim to have ONE day a week as a mini-fast to allow your body to carry on cleansing as much as possible so that the weight loss continues. Experiment with the suggested juices, smoothies and recipes and see what suits you best. Some people, like me, can't go to bed on an empty stomach, so if you are one of those, do a mini-fast from 8 in the morning to 8 at night. Or maybe from 4 in the afternoon to 4 the following afternoon will suit you better. It doesn't matter which hours you do your mini-fast as long as you give your body a 12-hour rest, once a week. You can do this throughout your long-term detox.

Quick detoxes – choose any of these

- One day a week have a 'live' food day only. Just fruit or just vegetables or a mixture of the two.
- Fast one day a week. Have lemon juice and hot water and vegetable juices only.
- Have a good breakfast, skip lunch and just have fruit in the evening.
- Have a half-day fast drinking one type of fruit juice, or vegetable juice, in the morning, followed by rice and vegetables and pulses in the evening.
- Eat one type of fruit or one type of vegetable ONLY all day.
- If you need more food: eat big raw salads with a little brown rice. You'll still detox.

One 'must have' supplement

Detoxil

As you read in the chapter on the liver, you can't detox properly on a low-protein diet as the liver needs essential amino acids (usually obtained from eating animal products such as meat, fish and eggs) to do its job properly. Amino acids are the building blocks of the body and cannot be manufactured within it.

The most vital amino acids for liver and kidney function are:

NAC – N-Acetyl cysteine – an antioxidant that breaks down mucus and neutralizes free radicals.

L-Glutathione – essential for Phase 2 of the liver's detoxification, an antioxidant that neutralizes free radicals so the toxins can be taken out of the body safely.

L-Methionine – an antioxidant that breaks down fat in the liver and is essential for the spleen, liver and pancreas to function properly.

These can be found in a supplement called Detoxil, which is an all-round detox support consisting of 26 bio-active nutrients, including: carotenoids, amino acids, vitamins C, E and vitamin B-complex plus natural diuretics dandelion and artichoke that work together to eliminate toxicity.

Other detox helpers included in Detoxil are: zinc for insulin metabolism, copper, iron, phosphatidylcholine for helping the liver break down fat, and grapefruit extract, which is an anti-fungal agent for a healthy bowel.

This is a good all-rounder that I would recommend to anyone, even if they are not following this plan, as it will help support your liver in its daily battle with toxins – especially if you live a stressful life, drink and smoke regularly and live in a city. Details of where to buy it can be found under Resources at the back of the book.

Recipes

Note on measurements

To simplify the recipes – so that you don't have to worry about weighing everything – I'm using a cup for larger measurements. This is the equivalent of about 250 ml – just under 9 fl oz (or just under ½ pint) and should represent the volume of a standard coffee mug.

Although the recipes are for one person, some of the measurements are more than generous, so that you can cook a dish that will feed you for more than one meal. If there are two of you, just double the ingredients.

LIVER FLUSH – SUGGESTED JUICE

It's important to repeat your liver flush juice whenever you can during your long-term detox. Here is a reminder of one of the best from the 48-Hour Kickstart Detox. But you can choose any of the other juices if you prefer.

The most important foods to help the liver detox are beetroot, radishes, watercress and ginger, because they help drain the liver by stimulating the gall bladder. If you can brave it, add one dessertspoon of olive oil to this juice because it is very high in phytonutrients, which benefit the liver, gall bladder and digestion. Or, if you prefer, you can use one of the Omega 3 or 6 oils. The garlic and cayenne pepper are both liver cleansers.

> 1 small beetroot
> 4 carrots
> 4 sticks of celery
> Handful of fresh watercress

6 radishes
Chunk of ginger
1–2 apples to sweeten
A squeeze of lemon

Optional
1 dessertspoon of olive oil or Omega 3 & 6 blended oil
2 teaspoons of freshly squeezed lemon juice
Pinch of cayenne pepper
1 clove of fresh garlic

LIVER CLEANSER FOR BLENDER

If you don't have a juicer, you can liquidize these ingredients in a blender instead:

200 ml organic apple juice
Juice of half a lemon with the pith
50–100 ml spring water
Pinch of cayenne
Pinch of ginger

Optional
1 tablespoon of olive oil or Omega 3 & 6 blended oil
1 clove of garlic

HOME-MADE HUMMUS

Hummus is generally made with chickpeas but as aduki beans are the most alkaline of the pulses and helpful for fluid elimination, try to make your hummus from aduki beans or the equally alkaline lima beans.

I have successfully made hummus with aduki beans and must admit, although it was a little mauve and 'windy', it was absolutely delicious. (I haven't found lima beans to date.) They're difficult to find ready cooked and canned so you will have to soak them for at least 4 hours and simmer them for another hour or so. Check the instructions on the packet. If you want an easier life, get ready-cooked pinto beans or chickpeas in a can.

> 1 standard can of cooked chickpeas, lima or aduki beans, drained
> Juice of one to two lemons (to taste)
> 1–2 teaspoons of tahini
> 2 cloves of garlic, crushed
> 1 tablespoon of tasteless flaxseed oil or hempseed oil
> 1 teaspoon of olive oil
> Parsley for decoration
> Good pinch of natural sea salt

STIR-FRY

> 1 packet of soya sausages
> Any amount of mixed vegetables, finely sliced
> Tamari
> Garlic
> Tomato paste
> Tahini paste

Chop up any carrots, broccoli and greens you have, or buy a pack of stir-fry vegetables, and fry the healthy way using stock or water first. Add flavourings such as Tamari and garlic, and a dessertspoon-ful of tahini paste to add some substance. Then add a packet of soya sausages chopped up into small pieces. You can add a drop of white wine, some tomato purée, anything that will add some flavour – as long as it's chemical-free. If you need more oil, you can add one of the 'healthy' Omega 3 oils at the end, once the pan is off the heat.

RATATOUILLE

My big pot version. Use any and as many vegetables as you like. I use carrots, broccoli, tomatoes, aubergine, peppers, green beans, tomato purée, garlic, and a little olive oil. Cook in a huge pot, very low and very long!

QUINOA

Quinoa is a wonderful protein-rich 'mother of all grains', but can taste a bit dull. David Smale, the owner and chef at my favourite restaurant in Brighton, The Coriander, gave this recipe to me – and it's delicious!

CORIANDER QUINOA

> 500 g quinoa
> 1 medium onion, finely diced
> 2–3 garlic cloves, finely diced
> 2–3 tablespoons of olive oil
> Smoked paprika
> 1 mild chilli, finely diced
> Vegetable stock – you'll need twice as much liquid as quinoa
>   (about 1 litre)
> Fresh coriander – finely chopped stalks, and leaves
> Seasoning

Put the quinoa in a frying pan and heat it gently, adding nothing, till it's golden. Remove. Sauté the onion, garlic, smoked paprika, chilli and seasoning. After 5 minutes, add chopped coriander stalks but not the leaves. Then add vegetable stock and the quinoa. Simmer for at least 15 minutes, till done. Just before serving, add finely chopped coriander leaves.

MIXED BEAN SALAD

> 400 g can of mixed beans
> Half red onion, finely chopped
> Parsley for decoration
> French dressing

This is a very quick and easy dish to prepare. Place the mixed beans in a dish, add the onions and the 'healthy' French dressing and decorate with parsley. Serve with a big green salad.

SUZI'S DRESSING

> 1 teaspoon of olive oil
> 2–3 tablespoons of Omega 3 & 6 oil
> 1 dessertspoon of cider vinegar
> 1 small clove of crushed garlic
> A very small teaspoon of mayonnaise
> Pinch of natural sea salt – I recommend Nature et Progrès
>   Seasalt

ADUKI BEANS WITH CREAMED AVOCADO DRESSING

Aduki beans are the most detoxifying of the pulses. In Chinese medicine they are the best for relieving water retention and good for the spleen. Avocado is full of vitamins, minerals and oils.

> 220 g tin of cooked aduki beans, drained and rinsed
> ½ cucumber
> 2 chopped tomatoes
> 1 stick of celery
> 1 spring onion
> Fresh basil and chives

AVOCADO DRESSING

(This can be used as a topping for any other dish)

> 2 small avocados
> 1 clove of garlic
> Lemon juice
> Tabasco
> Sea salt

Peel and de-stone the avocados. Pop into a blender and add the garlic, freshly squeezed lemon juice, a touch of Tabasco and a pinch of natural sea salt.

CHEAT'S MAYO

I cannot tell you how delicious this is and there isn't a trace of dairy in it. If you are missing your mayonnaise or creamy dressing and are going to eat a lot of salads, try this. Make sure you only use **silken** tofu or it is quite revolting!

> 1 teaspoon of capers
> 2 large cloves of crushed garlic
> 2 tablespoons of lemon juice
> ½ teaspoon of French mustard
> 1 tablespoon of brown rice vinegar or cider vinegar
> Tamari sauce
> 1–2 tablespoons of tasteless flaxseed oil
> 1 teaspoon of olive oil
> 275 g of silken tofu
> Soya milk or water to thin

Just combine all the ingredients in a blender and adjust for taste and texture.

AUBERGINE DIP

> One large aubergine
> Two tablespoons of freshly squeezed lemon juice
> 2 tablespoons of tasteless flaxseed oil
> 1 teaspoon of olive oil
> Chopped parsley
> 1 tablespoon of tahini
> 2 cloves of garlic
> Seasoning

Bake the aubergine in a pre-heated oven on 200°C, 400°F, gas mark 6. Bake until soft, 40–50 minutes. Cool then purée flesh in a blender with everything else. Chill.

BAKED VEGETABLES WITH BROWN RICE

> 1 yellow pepper
> 1 red pepper
> 1 orange pepper
> 1 aubergine
> Two courgettes
> Two red onions
> 6 tomatoes
> 3 small garlic cloves
> Seasoning: Nori flakes, Tamari
> Olive oil
> 1 portion of brown rice
> Hummus or tahini to taste

De-seed and slice the peppers, chop all the vegetables into small chunks and pop them into a big baking tin. Sprinkle with plenty of crushed garlic, Nori flakes and season with Tamari or a little natural sea salt. Drizzle olive oil all over and bake at medium heat till cooked and slightly brown. Usually about 45 minutes.

Once they are cooked, dress with lemon juice or a little cider vinegar and a little more olive oil. Leave them to cool in the marinade. Serve with brown rice and a dollop of hummus or tahini sauce on top.

BROWN RICE SALAD

Shiitake mushrooms are immune-boosting AND contain all 8 essential amino acids, so they are an excellent protein source.

> 1 cup of cooked brown rice
> 150 g shiitake mushrooms
> 4 tomatoes – chopped finely

1 chopped cucumber
4 spring onions, finely chopped
1 tablespoon of chopped parsley

Combine all of the ingredients and dress with Cheat's Mayo or Suzi's Dressing.

PENNY'S BAKED WINTER VEGETABLES

This is a delicious hot dish that T'ai Chi teacher Penny May suggested as an *occasional* meal during a long-term detox. It's a bit of a cheat as it is full of starchy root vegetables plus a little goat's cheese. But it's so tasty, and healthy, that it *has* to go in – especially if you're following this plan during the winter.

Four sweet potatoes, peeled and cubed
One small squash, peeled and cubed
Four large carrots, peeled and cubed
220 g can cooked chickpeas
220 g bag of spinach
Goat's cheese to garnish
Seasoning

Place the cubed potatoes, squash, and carrots in a baking tray and drizzle over a little olive oil. Cook in a medium oven till the vegetables are soft, about 30 minutes. Steam the spinach and add to the baking tray, along with the chickpeas and a little crumbled goat's cheese. Leave to cook for a further 5–10 minutes. And serve.

SAFFRON MILLET AND PUY LENTILS

275 ml cooked vegetable stock
110 g of puy lentils
110 g of millet
1–2 tablespoons of olive oil
1 leek, finely chopped
1 teaspoon cinnamon

2 cloves garlic, finely chopped

1 head of radicchio salad, shredded

Pinch of saffron threads or saffron powder

Add saffron to the stock and leave to soak for 10 minutes. Cook the lentils according to the instructions. Put millet in a frying pan and heat gently, adding nothing, till golden. Fry leek, garlic and cinnamon in a little olive oil for 3 minutes. Stir in lentils and millet and stock. Bring to boil and simmer for 30 minutes. Stir in radicchio at the end.

BROWN RICE AND CREAMED SPINACH

1 cup of uncooked brown rice

2 cups of vegetable stock

Olive oil

$\frac{1}{2}$ cup of chopped onions

1 cup of finely chopped celery

1 cup of sliced mushrooms

1 tablespoon of fresh herbs

1 cup of cooked, chopped spinach (can be from frozen)

$\frac{1}{2}$ cup of soy milk

Seasoning

Cook rice in stock and drain. In a little olive oil, sauté the rice, onions, celery, mushrooms and herbs. Combine spinach, soy milk, and seasoning in a blender and purée. Pour over rice mixture and serve with salad.

Healthy puds

NUT ICE CREAM

$\frac{1}{4}$–$\frac{1}{2}$ cup of mixed nuts and seeds

1 cup of vanilla soy milk

1 teaspoon of flaxseed oil

3 teaspoons of vanilla extract

Grind all the seeds and nuts, pop into the blender and add the milk, vanilla extract and oil. Blend till smooth. Pour into pudding glasses and pop into the freezer. Voilà, a healthy ice cream!

BANANA ICE CREAM

$\frac{1}{4}$ cup of blanched almonds
2 small bananas
Water

Blend the ingredients, pop into the freezer, and you have another healthy ice cream.

HEALTHY CAKE

(For visitors!)

2 cups of berries: blueberries, strawberries, raspberries or blackberries
6 cups of apple juice
1 tablespoon of vanilla extract
4 cups of millet or quinoa

Place juice, vanilla and grains in a large saucepan and bring to boil, stirring constantly until the grain has absorbed all the juices. Gently fold in the berries. Rinse a baking tin and leave it undried. Pour the mixture into the baking tin and place in fridge to chill and set. This will take about three hours. Then it should be ready to slice.

15.

Slimmer's Smoothies

Here is a reminder of the quiz you answered at the beginning of the book. Do the quiz again to see if your answers have changed since doing the Kickstart Detox weekend.

Slimmer's smoothies

> I have dry hair, scalp and skin
> My blood pressure is high
> I exercise regularly but can't lose weight
> I suffer from hormonal problems
> I need more energy
> I often get the blues
> I often feel tired and lethargic
> I suffer from skin problems such as acne and eczema
> My nails are very brittle and flaky
> I feel under the weather

More than 4 yeses – your body needs far more essential fatty acids than you are providing it with. During this plan you will be replacing TWO of your daily meals with a nutrient-packed and ridiculously filling smoothie that you make yourself in a blender. If you go out to work each day, you can have a smoothie for breakfast, a proper lunch as your main meal and a smoothie for supper. If you work at home you can have a smoothie for breakfast and one for lunch and have your main meal with your family in the evening.

Because the smoothie takes just 5 minutes to prepare, this plan will certainly suit those of you who live in the fast lane and prefer shakes or smoothies to sit-down meals. In fact, it was the perfect plan for me during the most productive part of writing this book because I didn't have to keep stopping to prepare meals. It will burn fat fast as well as bringing energy and health to every cell in your body.

You will also have one main, decent-sized meal a day. As long as you stick to the recommended foods in the recommended order of preference, you won't need to measure portions or calorie-count at all. It is an easy programme to follow, provided you have a blender and are strong-minded enough to follow the 'pyramid' below if eating away from home.

You will notice that the suggested foods for your main meals are very similar to those recommended in the next chapter, the high protein, low carbohydrate plan; those with the least sugar and starch.

Main meal – descending order of preferred foods for optimum weight loss

Green vegetables: salad greens, broccoli, asparagus, spinach, green beans, watercress, cabbage, fennel, kale etc.
Other vegetables: peppers, carrots, avocado, tomatoes etc.
Protein: oily fish, such as mackerel, salmon, herring, sardine and tuna, all other fish, chicken, turkey, eggs, soya, tofu, soya milk, and small amounts of goat's cheese & goat's milk.
Fruit: all berries, apples, kiwi, oranges, grapefruit, peaches, nectarines, mango, plums and fresh figs.
Seeds & Nuts: pumpkin & sunflower seeds, almonds, walnuts and macadamias etc. Almond milk.
Carbohydrates: oatmeal, millet, lentils, pulses, brown and wild rice, barley, rye, buckwheat, quinoa and rice milk.

As you can see, the foods that should make up the main proportion of your meals are at the top of the list, and foods such as fruit, seeds and nuts and carbohydrates should make up the *smallest* portion of your daily eating plan. Your main meal, in an ideal world, should be made up of plenty of greens and a light protein such as grilled chicken or fish. You can get even more EFAs into your system by using the French dressing from chapter 13's recipe suggestions. You'll find it repeated at the end of this chapter.

Keep carbohydrates to an absolute minimum, and choose only from those on the list. Try not to snack between meals. The smoothie is very filling and will give you all the nutrients, protein, fat and fibre you need to prevent you from feeling at all hungry.

Here is a reminder of the foods to avoid as far as you can:

Foods to eliminate or cut down on

Starchy carbohydrates – bread, potatoes, pasta, white rice, pastry etc

Biscuits, pastries, cakes, crisps, croissants etc

Cereals – apart from those made from the grains in the 'pyramid' list

Sweets, chocolate, and all sugar

Saturated fats – cheese, bacon, sausages and processed meat etc

Fried food

Fast food

Alcohol

Tea & coffee

Dairy – milk and cheese

Root vegetables, parsnips, corn, cooked carrots etc

'Sports' & soft drinks

All fruit *not* mentioned in the 'pyramid' list – in particular: melon, pineapple, orange *juice*, grapes, banana, and dried fruit, as they're very high in sugar

Red kidney beans & black-eye beans

Be aware of sauces, pickles, ketchup etc. They are all loaded with sugar, as is chewing gum, even if it's artificially sweetened. They all count.

This is the basis for any smoothie you might make for yourself during the programme, followed by a brief explanation as to why these ingredients are important and how they will help you fight the flab AND feel wonderful. You will find alternative smoothie recipes at the end of this chapter.

Smoothie ingredients

>   3–5 tablespoons of hempseed oil *and/or* flaxseed oil *or*
>   Omega 3 & 6 blended oil such as Udo's Choice
>   Unsweetened fruit juice – cranberry, apple, prune, grapefruit
>   etc
>   Fresh or frozen berries – strawberries, raspberries,
>   blueberries etc
>   *Or* a kiwi fruit
>   One tablespoon quark *or* cottage cheese *or* mixed nuts
>   1 heaped teaspoon to 1 dessertspoon of lecithin granules
>   One heaped dessertspoon 'Beyond Greens' from health
>   stores, see Resources
>   *Or* a heaped tablespoon of ground seeds
>   *And/Or* one glass of vegetable juice if you have a juicer
>   Rice, soya or almond milk if necessary

(You can substitute a ready-made shop-bought smoothie if short of time.)

Why fats can help you lose fat!

All fats, or lipids, are needed by the body to produce energy and to protect and insulate our vital organs. But it has to be the right kind of fat. We all know that saturated fats – cheese, lard, suet, bacon and fatty meats – will go straight on to our thighs and harden our arteries if eaten in excess.

But **essential** fats, in particular Omega 3 and 6, are a whole different ball game – especially Omega 3. Essential fatty acids are as essential to the body as calcium is to the bones and are so important for the health of every gland, organ and cell that your body won't waste them by laying them down as fat. In fact, you *can't* lose weight without them. Udo Erasmus, one of the world's leading experts on essential fats and author of *Fats that Kill, Fats that Heal*, says that EFAs will increase your metabolic rate, heat production, and energy levels, helping you to burn more calories, even at rest. 'Your body will go 40 times as far on fats as it will on carbohydrates,' says Erasmus. 'Omega 3 also turns on fat-burning in the body, and turns *off* fat production,' he adds.

EFAs also make you feel energetic so you are more likely to want to exercise and burn even more calories. They help your kidneys dump excess water held in your tissues and suppress your appetite as well as making your blood-sugar levels more stable, putting an end to cravings. Essential fats also play a very important role in brain health and their use in treating depression has been widely documented. If you feel happier you are less likely to overeat and more likely to feel like being active. I know these fats are 'happy' fats because none of my clients ever suffer from seasonal affective disorder when their diet is high in Omega 3 and 6.

A dozen reasons why EFAs are fat busters

1. Suppress appetite
2. Stop carbohydrate craving
3. Increase metabolism
4. Improve energy levels
5. Help oxygen into the cells
6. Improve thyroid function
7. Increase stamina
8. Burn more calories at rest
9. Help kidneys to dump excess water
10. Make you feel happy
11. Feed and protect friendly bowel bacteria
12. Slow down digestion

Essential fats

All EFAs must come from our food, we can't make them ourselves. But, because of our modern eating habits, most of us are seriously deprived of them – especially Omega 3. A daily diet rich in oily fish, seeds and nuts will probably deliver adequate amounts of Omega 3 and 6 for optimum health. But, for the purposes of the Slimmer's Smoothie programme, the best sources of Omega 3 and 6 are in oil form because you will be needing at least 6 tablespoons a day. Choose your oil wisely as you are going to get through quite a bit of it, so make sure it's one you like.

Flaxseed oil, also known as linseed oil

Flaxseed oil has the richest source of the essential fatty acid Omega 3 (alpha-linolenic acid). It also contains small amounts of Omega 6 (linoleic acid). But Udo Erasmus thinks flax oil is too high in Omega 3 in ratio to Omega 6 and recommends that you have a more balanced oil, such as Udo's Choice or hempseed oil. As you are going to need a lot of oil, especially if you are doing this in the middle of summer when less Omega 3 is needed, I tend to agree with him.

But if you like the taste of flaxseed oil you can use it quite safely in your smoothies by making sure you add either Omega 6-rich hempseed oil or lecithin granules.

Hempseed oil

Udo Erasmus considers hempseed oil to be nature's most perfectly balanced oil, due to its high content of *both* Omega 3 and Omega 6. It is readily available in most major supermarkets and health stores and seems, generally, to be more reasonably priced than flax oil.

Omega 3 and 6 blended oil

This takes all the work out of balancing the EFAs and you won't need to add lecithin to your smoothie.

Whether you buy flaxseed, hempseed or a blended Omega 3 and 6 oil, make sure you buy a good-quality oil that is cold-pressed and sold in a dark glass bottle. Oils oxidize very easily and can go rancid so keep it in the fridge AND DO NOT HEAT IT, or any other oil other than olive oil.

How much?

As Udo Erasmus and his son T'ai discovered when they worked with athletes and body builders, their clients were losing 5–15 lb a month of pure fat using as little as 3 and up to as much as 14 tablespoons of oil per day (whilst following a low-sodium, low-carbohydrate healthy diet). But the latter figure is a lot of oil!

For losing weight quickly and safely, and to turn you into a lean, mean, fighting machine, Udo recommends up to a *maximum* of 10 tablespoons a day for us ordinary mortals. That would be the equivalent of half your total calorie intake, which means you can't pig out when you sit down to your main meal of the day! However, the more tablespoons of oil you put in your smoothie, the less you should feel like eating because the oils suppress your appetite and make those carb cravings go away. The best barometer is to start on between 1 and 3 tablespoons in each smoothie and see how you feel. If you feel full of energy and your skin is soft and velvety you have ingested just the right amount and can work up to 5 table-spoons a smoothie.

But if you feel sick or suffer from any other symptoms, you have taken too much on an empty stomach and your liver is reacting. If you have done the detox, hopefully your liver will be OK. But if you are in any doubt at all, start with 2 tablespoons a smoothie and build up. Make sure you also use your preferred oil to drizzle over your main meal of the day to make up the quantity. And don't forget to check with a health professional if you are chronically ill, on medication or are at all concerned. Please don't follow this plan if you are pregnant.

One last warning – you may need less sleep when you start adding these oils to your diet in such large quantities. One of my clients complained that she couldn't get to sleep one night and couldn't understand it because she hadn't had any coffee at all, all day. I asked her what time she had drunk her smoothie and was told it was 9 p.m. You've been warned!

The great thing is, you really don't need to count calories using these fat-busting oils – just keep your intake of sugars, starches and saturated, non-essential fats to a minimum. That is why it's important to keep fruit, other than the fruit in your smoothie, and carbohydrates to a minimum while following this plan. Fruit and the listed starches are still a form of sugar, albeit the lowest form I could find.

How long?

Slimmer's Smoothies should work so quickly that you probably wouldn't need to follow this plan for more than a couple of weeks. You need to be the judge and jury at the end of the day. If you feel full of energy, full of food and the weight is coming off at a healthy and safe couple of pounds a week, then use the smoothies for as long as you need to and for as long as you can afford the oils. They cannot harm you, they can only do you good, but do please listen to your body and stop if you feel unwell or are losing weight too quickly.

Fruit juice

You can use any fruit juice you like for your smoothie, as long as it doesn't contain any added sugar. If you're really short of time, you can even buy a ready-made smoothie and keep it in the fridge. Some of the best ones are on sale in many places, from coffee shops to supermarkets, and include low-sugar, high-antioxidant berries such as blueberries and strawberries. Although not as nutritious as fresh fruit and juice, they still do the job.

If you have a juicer you may also like to do what I try to do once a day: add a glass of freshly juiced vegetables to the fruit base. This will deliver the biggest boost of fresh antioxidants and energy-giving nutrients you can give yourself in a glass. I juice whatever is lurking in the fridge till I have a small glass of vegetable juice. I then add it, along with the pulp from the juiced vegetables, to the blender before adding everything else to make up the smoothie. But you don't have to do this if you don't have the time. The rest of the ingredients in the smoothie will more than deliver all the nutrients and fibre your body needs.

There are suggestions for vegetable juices in chapter 13 and at the end of this chapter.

Why berries are best

There are several reasons why I always recommend berries for the smoothie recipe. Berries are extremely high in antioxidants and water, but very low in sugar. They are also more easily available in the frozen section should you be buying out of season. You only need a handful for each smoothie and, along with the lecithin granules, they have the capacity to turn an ordinary smoothie into a really delicious drink. You can also add any of the fruits recommended at the end of this chapter.

Protein

A tablespoon of quark or cottage cheese (both low-fat proteins) is recommended in each smoothie for several reasons. Protein is very important for supporting the liver and adrenals, so your body will function better first thing in the morning. This small amount of protein will also help fill you up, as it will make the smoothie more substantial.

But the most important reason for including this particular type of protein is because it interacts with the oil to give you even more energy. And remember – the more energy you have, the more weight you lose!

Dr Johanna Budwig, seven times Nobel prize nominee and considered to be one of the foremost authorities on fats and healing, recommends that essential fats should be put together with cottage cheese or quark because they both dissolve the oils more easily. When you mix one of the recommended oils with quark, cottage cheese or even nuts if you are a vegetarian, the amino acid cysteine in these proteins makes the fat become water-soluble, which makes it rich in electrons, carrying more energy and oxygen into your cells. Dr Budwig likens it to recharging a dead battery.

A quick lesson in electrons

As you know, the sun's rays reach the earth as a source of energy on which all the earth's minerals, plants and foods rely. The photon is the tiniest part of a sunbeam and is recognized as being the purest form of energy. Electrons love photons and are attracted to them much like we're attracted to chocolate! All the oils made from seeds (vegetable oils such as flax and hemp) are electron-rich and will help you absorb some of that sun's light and energy. This is why these oils are particularly important for any of us living in the Northern Hemisphere – especially in the winter when daylight hours are short.

Lecithin granules

If you are going to use flaxseed oil in your smoothie, because it is higher in Omega 3 than Omega 6 I would recommend you add lecithin granules because of their high Omega 6 content – they are 57 per cent Omega 6 to 7 per cent Omega 3. I would recommend lecithin even if you're not using flaxseed oil because it is such a good liver supporter and fills you up. More importantly, when you add lecithin granules to the smoothie, it acts like washing-up liquid, breaking down the fat, so the whole thing turns into a creamy, milk-shake-like drink with no trace of any oil.

Start with 1–3 heaped teaspoons of lecithin granules and build up to a dessertspoon if you like it and feel good on it. Some people need time for their livers to adjust to lecithin while others just love it. Just listen to your body and see how you feel. If you feel nauseous leave it out.

Lecithin granules can be found in any reputable health store.

'Beyond Greens'

The final product to add to your smoothie is another of my personal favourites because it takes all the work out of ensuring you get your daily quota of fibre, greens, seeds, antioxidants and digestive enzymes, all delivered in one heaped dessertspoon of green powder. Beyond Greens has been produced by Udo Erasmus and contains the following goodies:

- Carrots, soy sprouts, kale, bilberry and grape seed extract – antioxidants.
- Barley, alfalfa, oat and rye grasses, spirulina and chlorella – premium greens rich in all the vitamins and minerals we need.
- Flax, sunflower and sesame seeds – more EFAs
- Slippery elm, dulse, kelp and psyllium – detoxifying fibre for healthy bowels.
- Digestive enzymes – to help break down the food we're eating.

This wonderful green powder will provide all the bulk you need in your smoothie. You will not go hungry if you add one heaped dessertspoon per smoothie and it will help balance your blood-sugar levels at that time of the day when you generally reach for coffee or a chocolate bar. There are many similar products in health stores so have a look around and make sure any product you buy includes a high proportion of greens, fibre and nutrients.

If you prefer you can, instead, grind up sunflower, flax and pumpkin seeds to make up a heaped *tablespoon* and also add a heaped *teaspoon* of psyllium husks to the smoothie, as well as juicing your own vegetables. This would give you a similar concoction but would obviously take more preparation.

So that's the run-down of the powerful ingredients that will go into your Slimmer's Smoothies. I'm sure you'll agree, once you've had a chance to experiment and find your favourite combination, that the smoothies are filling, satisfying and quite delicious. To end this chapter, here are some suggestions for main meals and smoothies – just whiz up any of the following in a blender.

NUTTY NECTARINE

> 3–5 tablespoons of hempseed and/or flaxseed or Omega
>   3 & 6 blended oil such as Udo's Choice
> Small glass of unsweetened apple & mango juice
> Handful of fresh or frozen raspberries
> 1 nectarine
> 1 tablespoon of quark or cottage cheese or mixed nuts
> Three heaped teaspoons of lecithin granules
> One heaped dessertspoon of Beyond Greens
> 1 small glass of almond milk

BLUEBERRY BLUFF

> 3–5 tablespoons of hempseed and/or flaxseed or Omega
>   3 & 6 blended oil such as Udo's Choice
> Small glass of unsweetened prune juice
> Handful of blueberries
> 1 peach
> 1 tablespoon of quark or cottage cheese or mixed nuts
> Three heaped teaspoons of lecithin granules
> 1 heaped dessertspoon of Beyond Greens
> 1 small glass of almond or rice milk

THREE BERRIES

> 3–5 tablespoons of hempseed and/or flaxseed or Omega
> 3 & 6 blended oil such as Udo's Choice
> Small glass of unsweetened apple juice
> Handful of mixed berries: strawberries, raspberries, and
> loganberries
> 1 tablespoon of quark or cottage cheese or mixed nuts
> Three heaped teaspoons of lecithin granules
> 1 heaped dessertspoon of Beyond Greens or ground
> seeds
> 1 small glass of sweetened soya milk

TANGY TANGERINE

> 3–5 tablespoons of hempseed and/or flaxseed or Omega
> 3 & 6 blended oil such as Udo's Choice
> Small glass grapefruit juice
> 1–2 tangerines, de-pipped
> Half a mango
> 1 tablespoon quark or cottage cheese, or mixed nuts
> Three heaped teaspoons of lecithin granules
> 1 heaped dessertspoon of Beyond Greens
> 1 teaspoon of a sugar substitute if necessary: Valdivia sugar,
> brown rice sugar or date sugar

VEGETABLE-BASED SMOOTHIE

Juice your favourite vegetables and add to your chosen fruit
smoothie, with or without the pulp.

> 2 apples
> 3 carrots
> 1 small beetroot
> 1 chunk of red cabbage
> 2 sticks of celery

Handful of watercress
Handful of alfalfa sprouts
Piece of ginger to taste

Main meal suggestions

Here's a reminder of the salad dressing from chapter 13 which is rich in Omega 3 & 6 EFAs, to help you to make up your quota of a *maximum* of 10 tablespoons a day. You can drizzle this over any salads you have with your protein main meal.

SUZI'S DRESSING

1 teaspoon of olive oil
2–3 tablespoons of flaxseed or hempseed oil, or blended oil
1 dessertspoon of cider vinegar
1 small clove of crushed garlic
A very small teaspoon of mayonnaise
Pinch of natural sea salt – I recommend Nature et Progrès
   Seasalt

Fish dishes

One serving of smoked mackerel or grilled salmon with
   rocket salad
Fresh tuna with steamed asparagus and salad
Smoked salmon with a big green salad, one piece of rye
   bread
Tinned tuna with watercress served on rye or buckwheat
   bread
Grilled sardines with a big green salad
Any other fish, grilled and served with steamed green
   vegetables or a salad and a little brown or wild rice
Kippers with grilled tomatoes and mushrooms
Salad niçoise without the potatoes

Eggs & cheese

Mushroom and tomato omelette with a big green salad
Grilled goat's cheese (one small portion) on rocket salad,
    with 2 oatcakes
Egg mayonnaise
Greek feta salad

Meat

Chicken with grilled peppers and salad, a small portion of
    brown rice
Cooked chicken or turkey with broccoli, spinach or green
    beans, a tiny portion of potatoes
Venison or partridge or any 'wild' meat with red cabbage,
    braised fennel and kale, wild rice
Turkey salad – any combination of vegetables from the list
Coronation chicken salad
Caesar salad without the cheese

Vegetarian suggestions

Soya sausages, grilled, with tomatoes, mushrooms and
    served with rocket
A whole avocado with a big green salad, grated carrots,
    beetroot and a tablespoon of hummus
Tofu burger with salad
Baked beans on rye bread
Grilled vegetables with a small portion of brown basmati rice
    and a tahini dressing (see chapter 13 recipes)

Snacks

Half a grapefruit
2 plums
1 orange or tangerine

One apple, peach or nectarine
A small handful of mixed seeds
A small handful of mixed nuts
2 oatmeal biscuits with a thin layer of hummus or goat's
cheese
1 boiled egg
Half an avocado

Drinks

Don't forget to drink water – at least 2 litres a day
Green tea, herbal tea, or a cup of miso broth
One cup of organic tea or coffee a day – if you must!

If you are eating out – pyramid

This is the pyramid of foods that you should be eating: the largest
portion of the meal should be green vegetables, followed by other
vegetables, then by protein. The oils should be supplying half of
your daily calorie intake so keep carbohydrates, other fats and fruit
to an absolute minimum at your main meal. Concentrate on just
protein and green vegetables wherever possible and the pounds will
fly off you!

Have another look at the quiz you answered at the beginning of the
chapter. If you have followed the Slimmer's Smoothie programme
for at least two weeks, all of the statements below should be a thing
of the past. Hopefully, you now have lovely velvety skin, happy
hormones AND you've lost weight!

I have dry hair, scalp and skin
My blood pressure is high
I exercise regularly but can't lose weight
I suffer from hormonal problems
I need more energy
I often get the blues

I often feel tired and lethargic
I suffer from skin problems such as acne and eczema
My nails are very brittle and flaky
I feel under the weather

The great thing about this weight-loss plan is that you can go back to it whenever you like. If you've returned to eating two meals a day, you can make your third meal a Slimmer's Smoothie, using 1–2 tablespoons of oil instead of 5, and still reap the benefits of these magic oils, without regaining any weight. If you feel you need to lose more weight, you can go back to the plan whenever you like. The smoothies are so quick, nutritious and easy to prepare it makes life a lot simpler for those of us who don't have a spare 5 minutes to prepare a meal.

There is one final reminder. As you may have read earlier, successful weight loss relies on synergy – 'the working together of two or more components to be more successful or productive as a result of a merger'. In other words, you need more than two components in order to lose weight successfully.

You now know what not to eat to keep the weight off, but please don't forget the other two components: exercise and the emotional level – the link between the mind and the body.

If you have all three components in place, you cannot fail to reach your optimum weight. Here's a final reminder of what you need to continue to do to get all three components working together:

CONTINUE AS MUCH AS POSSIBLE:

Tibetan 5 rites – these are muscle-toning and energizing exercises, so try and continue them each day. It will only take you 5 minutes and will set you up for the day.
Skin-brushing – every day before your shower this will clear away any toxicity and dead cells that have gathered on your skin overnight.
Two litres of water a day – you can't lose weight without nature's diuretic and it will fill you up.

Four hours of exercise a week – this is essential if you really want to burn fat. It doesn't matter what you do, as long as you do it!

Sauna – this is very beneficial on this weight-loss programme. It has been found that oil-soluble toxins will leave the body in the oil part of the sweat – so the more you sweat the more you get rid of waste. Waste = weight!

Your favourite affirmation or technique from the weekend – choose an exercise you particularly liked during the Kickstart Detox and practise it daily.

16.

High-Protein Diet, Low-Carb

Here is a reminder of the quiz you answered at the beginning of the book. Do the quiz again to see if your answers have changed since doing the Kickstart Detox weekend.

High-protein, low-carb

> I feel very groggy in the morning
> I feel irritable if I miss a meal
> I have a family history of adult-onset diabetes
> I often crave alcohol, cigarettes or coffee
> I crave chocolate regularly
> I crave starchy foods such as bread, bananas and potatoes
> I have no time to prepare special meals
> I eat out regularly
> I suffer the afternoon slumps
> I often eat when I'm not hungry

More than 4 yeses – you need this weight-loss plan to improve your blood-sugar levels. This is the easiest plan to follow for anyone living in the real world. Whether you're a frantic mum with a family or a busy executive who eats out all the time, you should find this plan really simple to follow. Blood-sugar-level problems, insulin resistance, a sluggish thyroid and even Candida symptoms should vanish on this plan. (If you know you are a Candida sufferer, there is a separate list of foods you should avoid in the 'What to eat, What not to eat' section on page 187.)

This is such a safe and healthy high-protein, low-carb eating plan that I follow it myself as well as putting a great number of my clients on it. It fits in with their busy lifestyles and their weight loss is steady, painless and permanent. The only people who find this plan a little difficult to follow are vegans and vegetarians. I have included a choice of non-animal proteins for you in the 'What to eat, What not to eat' section.

Why high-protein/low-carb?

Nowadays, high-protein, low-carbohydrate 'diets' are rarely out of the news. Especially the NO carbohydrate diets that allow as much saturated fat as you like. You know the ones: fried bacon and eggs for breakfast, ham and cheese for lunch, steak and eggs for dinner. There is no doubt that these diets work, in the short term. But no one knows the long-term health implications of following them. An excess of protein can cause a complete imbalance in the body's mineral deposits and acid/alkaline balance, leading to kidney stones, liver problems and weaker bones. You may think you're getting plenty of calcium from all that cheese, but an excess of protein is causing calcium to be literally leached out of the bones. A complete absence of fibrous vegetables and fruit can also cause constipation, bowel problems and bad breath!

But a high-protein diet, that works, doesn't have to mean NO carbs and a load of unpleasant side effects. On this plan, you are going to have plenty of green vegetables (high in fibre and carbohydrate). You'll also be eating plenty of energy-giving protein and fat-busting fats. You won't go hungry, you *will* lose weight and, most importantly, you'll improve your long-term health.

Why carbs can put on weight

Believe it or not, high-protein, low-carbohydrate diets have been fashionable since the time of Hippocrates (500 BC). That long ago, diets high in protein and fat and low in carbohydrates were recommended for those who needed to reduce their body fat.

Much more recently many practitioners, including the late Dr Atkins, decided that most overweight people have got that way because their bodies aren't metabolizing carbohydrates properly.

But why all of a sudden? Haven't we been eating grains and starches all our lives? Actually, we haven't! Millions of years ago we kept strong and healthy by eating the fish and game we caught, and plenty of seeds, nuts, fruit and vegetables in between. There was ample carbohydrate in all those foods to give us enough energy to hunt all day – by foot.

It was only when we stopped being hunter-gatherers and became farmers, a few thousand years ago, that we began eating wheat and other grains. Professor Loren Cordain, from the Department of Health and Exercise Science at Colorado State University, thinks this is when our problems began. The human body just didn't have time to evolve, according to Cordain.

I think there's an additional reason why carbs and starches are being blamed for everything from gut problems to insulin resistance and weight gain. We eat too much of them for the amount of energy we're using and most of them – especially refined carbo-hydrates – are stashed full of additives, preservatives, salt and sugar. They've moved away from their natural state as far as it's possible to get.

Carbohydrates *are* good fuels, but if you eat more than you need, your body transforms the excess into fat and stores it for later. Body fat is simply a form of energy storage. You are literally wearing your excess fuel, waiting for the next famine! If you *decrease* carbs and *increase* exercise those fat reserves are converted straight back to fatty acids for the body to use as fuel.

Don't forget that certain starches can also make you feel heavy and look three months pregnant because every single unit of glyco-gen your body produces from that starch needs three times as much water to store it. Every wholemeal sandwich you eat needs three glasses of water to convert the starch to glycogen which, for many of us, results in a swollen tummy.

Finally, I have put a good three quarters of my own clients on a high-protein, low-carbohydrate eating plan because so many of them are suffering from rampaging blood-sugar levels, and are well on their way to becoming insulin-resistant. If you had more than four yeses in answer to the quiz at the beginning of this chapter, you too could be suffering from the blood-sugar blues. Don't panic, it's not a serious problem and is easily sorted if it's nipped in the bud now.

Insulin resistance & the blood-sugar blues

If I told you that you couldn't have hot buttered toast for the next three weeks how would you react? If the idea of living without toast, pasta, bread or bananas fills you with absolute HORROR, the odds are that you are on your way to becoming insulin-resistant. Especially if you are carrying an unexplained spare tyre around your middle and suffer from those awful late-afternoon sugar blues when nothing but chocolate will do. Don't worry, you're not alone. Our 21st-century eating habits – a diet high in sugar, stimulants and refined carbohydrates – has led to an epidemic of blood-sugar problems, insulin resistance, obesity and adult-onset diabetes. We've all turned into 'carb junkies' and our health is suffering because of it.

Funny, isn't it? Loads of us are addicted to hot buttered toast, but not many of us are addicted to greens! Don't worry, you will be. I used to eat pasta every night and sandwiches every day. I now have pasta about twice a year, bread about twice a month and yes I do, now, crave greens. Your body changes once your blood-sugar levels are sorted out and this eating plan will sort them out once and for all.

Insulin production & blood sugars

From the carbohydrates you eat, your body will absorb simple sugars into its bloodstream, which it will then turn into glucose. The glucose is converted to glycogen to store in your muscles and liver for energy. IF the glycogen stores are full and there is still more glucose coming in, the excess will be converted straight to triglycerides – fat, to you and me.

The more refined carbs you eat, the more insulin the pancreas has to produce. The more it produces, the less efficient the body becomes at converting glucose into energy and the **more is stored as fat**. Eventually, when the pancreas becomes so exhausted from being asked, repeatedly, to produce more insulin, insulin resistance sets in. It just can't keep up any more.

Stress, forgetting to eat, and living on stimulants such as sugar, nicotine, caffeine and alcohol can also all contribute to raging blood-sugar levels. Every time we grab that extra cup of coffee or second chocolate bar, the level of glucose in the blood surges and so do our energy levels – temporarily. The pancreas produces more insulin to stabilize the glucose levels and the energy high is followed, swiftly, by an energy low. This brings on tiredness, lethargy, irritability or a headache. Eventually, these blood-sugar highs and lows will exhaust our adrenals, as well as the pancreas, making us exhausted, foggy-headed, moody and water-retentive. Just check this list to see if it rings any bells.

Further signs of insulin resistance & blood-sugar problems

Needing to nibble between meals
Needing a cigarette to get going
Bingeing on things you crave
Not able to get going in the morning without coffee
Starving by supper
Gobbling food down
Feeling low for no reason
Suffering from seasonal affective disorder
Sensitive to light

Glycaemic index

So, if you want to lose weight and balance your blood-sugar levels, it is important to become aware of the foods that release blood sugar very fast. The higher a food is on the glycaemic index, the GI, (and it varies from expert to expert) the faster it releases sugar into the bloodstream and the more it's going to affect you and your blood-sugar levels.

If you are a 'carb junkie', many of the foods on the Bad Carbs list will be very familiar friends to you. Make a decision now that you CAN live without your friends for a few weeks. You'll appreciate them so much more when your weight has fallen off and your energy levels have gone sky high. And you'll be amazed at how infrequently you'll need to see them again, once you've got used to living without them on a daily basis!

Seemingly healthy food such as mashed potato, which actually appears high on the glycaemic index, can release sugar into the bloodstream almost as fast as sweets or chocolate. Low GI foods, such as protein, release sugar slowly into the blood in quantities the body can cope with. Energy is sustained over a much longer time and blood-sugar highs and lows become a thing of the past.

To make it simple, the lists are divided into the good, the bad and the OK carbs or starches. Don't forget even vegetables and fish have a certain amount of carbohydrate in them so you won't be going without your carbs.

What not to eat

Bad carbs

Alcohol	Biscuits
Sugar	Pastry
Cakes	Coffee
White Rice	Cooked Carrots
Tea	Corn
Maize	Honey
Crisps	Sweets
Chocolate	Glucose
Melon	French Fries
Pineapple	White Pasta
Grapes	White Bread
Bagels	Mashed Potato
Cornflakes	Baked Potato

Cereals	Croissant
'Sports' Drinks	Parsnips
Soft Drinks	Orange Juice
Sweet Potato	Shredded Wheat/Weetabix
Popcorn	Red Kidney Beans
Black-Eye Beans	Split Peas
Banana	Raisins
Dried Fruit	Haricot Beans
Milk	Couscous
Pears	Prunes

Be aware of sauces, pickles, ketchup etc. They are all loaded with sugar, as is chewing gum, even if it's artificially sweetened. They all count as bad carbs.

What to eat

OK carbs 2–3 times a week

Avocado	Eggs
Barley	Amaranth
Buckwheat	Beetroot
Oats	Porridge
Wholegrains	Sweetcorn
Sesame Seeds	Sunflower Seeds
Oatmeal Biscuits	Brown Basmati Rice
Kiwi Fruit	Pumpernickel Bread
Baked Beans	Oranges
Apple Juice	Apples
Root Vegetables	Muesli (unsweetened)
Plums	Rye
Spelt	Millet
Quinoa	

Good carbs

Alfalfa Sprouts	Artichoke
Asparagus	Broccoli
Celery	Chicory
Courgettes	Cucumber
Salad Leaves	Fennel
French Beans	Kale
Leeks	Onions
Mushrooms	Parsley
Peas	Spinach
Cauliflower	Tomatoes
Olives	Watercress
Chicken	Fish
Tofu	All fowl
Lentils	Pulses
Pumpkin Seeds	Flaxseeds
Chickpeas	Raw Goat's Milk
Soya Milk	Cherries
Nuts	Berries
Grapefruit	Raw Carrots (1–2 daily)
Peaches	Nectarines

For maximum energy and weight loss, you need to avoid the foods on the bad carbs list as much as you can. Eat the OK carbs in moderation and eat as much as you like, with a couple of exceptions, of the foods on the good carbs list.

To make it even simpler, here is a list of the perfect daily foods to eat, in descending order of importance. As in all the other plans, green vegetables are top of the tree but grains are way down at the bottom. This is your key to healthy weight loss, healthy adrenals and insulin levels, improved energy levels and faster weight loss. There will be meal suggestions at the end of this chapter.

Perfect daily foods in descending order

Green vegetables

Raw vegetable juice

Other vegetables from the OK and good lists

Mushrooms – a small portion, 75 g, daily

Peppers – red, yellow or green. One a day

Oily fish – tuna, mackerel, salmon, herrings & sardines etc

Seeds, nuts & olives – a maximum of 20 g a day

Essential fatty acids – flaxseed or hempseed oil – 1
     tablespoon daily

All other fish – grilled or baked

Poultry – chicken, turkey, pheasant, partridge etc

Meat – venison, rabbit, wild boar, buffalo – anything wild
     and free-range

Red meat – very occasionally treat yourself to steak or lamb
     chops

Eggs – 2–3 a week

Quark, cottage cheese or 'live' yoghurt – 1 tablespoon daily

Goat's cheese, mozzarella, halloumi (all non-cow cheeses) –
     equivalent to a heaped tablespoon, 2–3 times a week

Fruit – 1–2 portions daily

A *little* butter, cream or sour cream – in very small amounts
     these are not *bad* fats

Grains from OK and good list – 2–3 times a week, a small
     portion

A small glass of dry wine – 2–3 a week, maximum

Green vegetables

As in all the previous plans, the emphasis is on green vegetables,
raw wherever possible. People forget that all vegetables are actually
complex carbohydrates, full of fibre. So, unless you are an athlete
training for a marathon or someone who exercises for more than
two hours a day, a plateful of greens will give you all the carbo-

hydrate your body needs. Greens are also the highest in nutrients and poorest in calories so deserve to be top of the tree.

Raw vegetable juice

A vegetable juice should be part of this eating plan not only for the benefits of a nutrient-packed drink but also because high-protein diets can cause ketosis. When the body starts breaking down fat (which it will in the absence of carbohydrates) ketones are produced and excreted via your urine. This can make you feel tired, headachy, constipated and give you bad breath. You won't get any of these symptoms if you eat your greens and/or incorporate a vegetable juice each day, using vegetables from the OK and good lists. If you are out and about, you can always buy a ready-made bottle of vegetable juice. It's not as rich in fresh vitamins and minerals but will help prevent ketosis.

Other vegetables

You will notice that root vegetables (with the exception of baked and mashed potato) are only recommended 2–3 times a week because they are quite starchy. (Baked and mashed potatoes are on the bad list and should be excluded altogether because they are too high in sugar to be eaten regularly.) I have made raw carrots and beetroot the two exceptions because they are so good for you in a juice or grated on salads. So by all means have these two superfoods daily but keep strictly to 1–2 carrots a day and no more than half a small beetroot. Always have them raw because cooking starchy vegetables releases the sugar they contain and will push them higher up the glycaemic index and make them a no-no.

Don't OD on mushrooms or peppers either, as they are also quite starchy.

Oily fish & other healthy fats

Salmon, tuna, sardines, mackerel and herring – as you now know – are full of the essential fats Omega 3 and 6. These EFAs are essential for the health of every cell in your body and are top of the pops when it comes to weight loss. You can eat a portion of oily fish every single day if you like.

Seeds and nuts – particularly almonds, brazils, walnuts and macadamias – are also very healthy, protein-rich fats which, again, are essential for your health and wellbeing, providing Omega 3 essential fats to suppress your appetite and speed up your metabolism. Unless you are a vegetarian, don't have more than 20 g a day as you'll be getting more than enough protein and essential fats from your fish. If you don't like oily fish at all, you can eat larger portions of seeds and nuts.

Despite their reputation for being 'fattening', olives and avocados are also very healthy fats – in moderation. Have no more than half a dozen olives at a time and avocados two to three times a week only.

The other reason I'm a fan of avocado is because it contains the enzyme lipase, which prevents the fat we consume from being stored. Lipase is found in all high-fat 'live' foods, such as 'live' yoghurt and seeds and nuts. So I've put all these foods into the OK and good carbs list because they're so good for you.

Essential fats

Essential fats are still the best way to re-programme your cells to burn fat. They are also essential because they will suppress your appetite, balance your blood-sugar levels and hormones, speed up your metabolism and help you lose weight.

Essential fatty acids, found in Omega 3 & 6 oils, are also essential for protein metabolism and will help prevent your system from becoming too acidic. Make sure you have at least one tablespoon of flaxseed, hempseed oil or a blended oil a day. Put it into your salad dressing or drizzle over your food. DO NOT HEAT IT.

Fish, meat, eggs and fowl

Protein foods such as meat, fish and tofu contain little or no carbohydrate and therefore cannot upset your blood-sugar levels. In fact, quite the contrary, as the glucagon produced by protein helps to stabilize blood-sugar levels.

If you don't like oily fish, there are plenty of alternatives you can eat, including all shellfish, white fish and any fish you like as long as it's not fried. (But make sure to have one tablespoon of oil a day for your EFAs.)

If you're a meat-eater, try to buy organic, free-range and 'wild' meat wherever possible. Vension, rabbit, wild boar, buffalo and of course chicken, turkey and pheasant can now be found in quite a few organic stores and supermarkets and are more likely to have been grass-fed and more naturally reared. More importantly, they contain less saturated fat and are a healthier alternative to red meat.

If your budget doesn't run to the more 'exotic' meats, go ahead and have lamb chops, steak or pork, occasionally. This isn't your cue to eat as much meat as you like and to start each day with steak and eggs. Even if the red meat you buy is organic, it is still a very 'acidic', saturated fat, and can cause bone and kidney problems if eaten in excess.

Eggs really are a meal in themselves, so please do go ahead and have an omelette, scrambled or poached eggs several times a week.

Quark, cottage cheese or 'live' yoghurt

I've included the above three dairy products because quark and cottage cheese are both very low in fat and very high in protein. 'Live' yoghurt is also high in lipase, an essential enzyme for fat prevention, as well as good bacteria to promote a healthy bowel. Allow yourself one heaped tablespoon a day of your preferred dairy product.

Goat's cheese, mozzarella & halloumi cheese

Life can be very dull without cheese so I have included three that are non-dairy, lower in saturated fat than cow's cheese and tasty enough to satisfy those cheese urges. There are all sorts of goat's cheeses on sale in supermarkets now, ranging from feta to Camembert and Gouda. Mozzarella cheese can be made from either cow's milk or buffalo milk, so look for one made from buffalo milk, as it will be lower in saturated fat. Halloumi cheese is usually made from ewe's milk and although very salty, it's still not dairy and is delicious marinated in pesto and well worth a try. But don't go mad, try to stick to the equivalent of one heaped tablespoon 2–3 times a week only.

Fruit – one portion daily

You may be surprised to find fruit so low down the 'pyramid', despite its health benefits. Although fruit is full of antioxidants, vitamins and minerals it is also very high in sugar – albeit natural sugar. Vegetables are a much better source of nutrients and are much lower in starch and natural sugar, so keep fruit to a minimum and make it one or two pieces a day.

 TOP TIP

Raspberries and strawberries are the lowest in the sugar stakes, but you can have any fruit from the OK and good list, in moderation.

Bad fats you can eat

A little butter, cream and sour cream

Contrary to popular belief, the most dangerous fats are found in margarines, heated oils and 'hydrogenated' products. They produce trans-fatty acids that function differently from more natural fats in the body. Butter, on the other hand, may be a saturated fat but it is also high in vitamin A and vitamin D and made completely *naturally* from whole milk. A *little* butter is better for you than any other spreads or margarines.

The same applies to cream, sour cream and mayonnaise. The odd couple of teaspoons aren't going to hurt you as long as you buy FULL-fat rather than LOW-fat products. Anything low-fat has had most of the goodness taken out and often has salt, sugar, colourings or additives put back in to make it tastier. Check the labelling carefully, and have a little of the most *natural* fat you can find. If you have enough fat in your diet you won't end up hungry all the time, desperate to snack on starchy carbs such as chocolate and biccies. So have a little of what you fancy – in moderation.

Grains – a small portion daily if needed

Quinoa, spelt, oats, brown basmati rice, rye & millet are the best grains to eat, as they are extremely high in protein and low in starch. (Brown basmati rice is lower in starch than plain brown rice.)

These grains would also be very useful for vegetarians following this plan because when they are mixed with tofu or pulses the meal becomes a complete-protein meal, delivering all eight of the essential amino acids needed by your body.

For the rest of you, especially in the winter when you'll need more bulk, by all means have these grains when you want them, but always make sure they make up the very *smallest* proportion of your meal.

Pulses, lentils, hummus etc are NOT recommended for any non-vegetarians following this plan as they are equally high in carbohydrate and protein and you will be getting more than enough protein from the animal products you'll be eating. Vegetarians and vegans can go ahead and eat pulses for the valuable protein they supply.

Alcohol

A small glass of booze – 2–3 a week, maximum.

I bet that caught your attention! I will leave the number of glasses a week up to you, but if you are going to follow this plan for longer than a couple of weeks you will find it very difficult to dine out and go to functions without joining in with the occasional glass of wine. You know alcohol is almost pure sugar and is, strictly speaking, a carbohydrate high on the 'baddies' list. But if you really can't avoid it, try to keep it to one or two glasses a week. Avoid beer and wine unless it's very dry and, wherever possible, try to drink neat vodka or tequila instead as they both contain less sugar and are a purer form of alcohol.

For vegetarians

Vegetarians and vegans need to make sure to get plenty of protein and protein-rich meals by mixing pulses, nuts and seeds *with* the grains. As you will see from the following list, you can have much bigger portions of pulses, nuts and seeds than your meat-eating colleagues can.

Don't forget that quinoa and millet are extremely high-protein grains, so I would put them top of your grains tree if I were you. A good example would be stir-fried quinoa pieces (on sale in many health stores) or tofu pieces with millet. Or grilled vegetables with brown basmati rice and a generous dollop of hummus.

> Tofu or quorn – any amount – burgers, sausages, rissoles etc
> Pulses – 50 g a day
> Nuts – 150 g a day
> Eggs – one DAILY
> Cheese – stick to non-cow wherever possible
> Anything else you like from the OK and good lists

Pulses

Chickpeas	Black-eye Beans
Pinto Beans	Lentils
Flageolet Beans	Split Peas
Kidney Beans	Soy Beans

Finally, if you suffer from **Candida**, here is a list of foods – in addition to the 'bad' carbs – you should avoid for a minimum of 3 weeks but preferably 6 weeks. You can then start reintroducing a 'baddie' one at a time, leaving a gap of four days before eating it again or reintroducing another food.

You should have greatly improved symptoms following the high-protein, low-carb diet, provided you eliminate sugar, and yeasty and fermented foods as much as possible. You might also like to take 2 teaspoons of a colon cleanser daily, to ensure healthy bowel bacteria, which is essential if you are to win your battle against Candida albicans.

Eliminate

Cheese	Fruit
Mushrooms	Spicy Food
Vinegar (except organic cider vinegar)	Coffee
	Peanuts
Dried Fruits	Soy Sauce
Wine	Yams
Beer	Sweet Potatoes

In moderation, intermittently

Miso	Nuts
Tempeh	Seeds
Tofu	Avocados

Two essential supplements

There are two secret weapons to consider if you want to follow this plan – lecithin and a digestive enzyme. Protein can be very hard to digest and undigested food can sit in your colon for days, fermenting and causing toxicity. A digestive enzyme will help your body break down protein and make the nutrients from it more absorbable. It does your digestion's work for you.

So take a digestive enzyme with every meal whilst you are following any high-protein, low-carbohydrate programme. Try and find one in capsule form and, ideally, sprinkle it over hot food. This will give better results than just swallowing it with your meal. 1–2 digestive enzymes are recommended for each meal and any brand will do. If you are over 40, make sure your supplement contains hydrochloric acid, or bromelain, as these enzymes are more difficult for the body to produce naturally as you get older.

If you are going to eat more fat than normal, in the shape of cheese, cream and other fats, I would also recommend that you take 'fat-loving' lecithin granules to help protect your cholesterol levels. Take a couple of heaped teaspoons a day.

Meal suggestions

Breakfast

> Grilled kippers with tomatoes and mushrooms
> Smoked salmon and a little quark or cottage cheese on one slice of rye or pumpernickel bread
> 1 poached egg with mushrooms and tomatoes
> A vegetable juice: 2 carrots, 3 sticks of celery, 1 small apple, and a handful of watercress, alfalfa sprouts and a small piece of ginger
> Slimmer's Smoothie as in chapters 13 & 15, sticking to fruit from the OK & good list only
> Baked beans with tomatoes and mushrooms
> Half a grapefruit with a small handful of pumpkin seeds

Oat-based muesli with goat's or soya milk – a small bowl
One portion of fruit with one tablespoon of 'live' yoghurt
(cow's, goat's or sheep's yoghurt)
Soya sausages, mushrooms and tomatoes

For extra Omega 3, make salad dressing using flaxseed, hempseed, or blended Omega 3 & 6 oil, instead of olive oil. You can't lose weight without Omega 3 & 6 but you *can* put weight on using large amounts of olive oil.

SUZI'S DRESSING

1 teaspoon of olive oil
2–3 tablespoons of Omega 3 & 6 oil
1 dessertspoon of cider vinegar
1 small clove of crushed garlic
Pinch of natural sea salt – I recommend Nature et Progrès
Seasalt
1 small teaspoon of mayonnaise

Lunch

Baked salmon with a big green salad or spinach
Prawn cocktail with half an avocado
Grilled goat's cheese on rocket salad
Grilled chicken with green vegetables or salad
Tinned tuna salad niçoise: green beans, egg, salad, pepper,
olives but NO potatoes
Omelette and salad
Egg mayonnaise
Artichoke with French dressing
Mozzarella, tomatoes, olives and basil
Greek salad: feta cheese, olives, tomatoes, cucumber and
salad leaves

Supper

Grilled sardines and any vegetables from the good carbs list

Turkey salad or roast turkey with broccoli, green beans and fennel

Smoked mackerel with salad

Halloumi cheese marinated overnight in pesto, grilled and served with salad

Venison, chicken or pheasant with red cabbage and broccoli

Fish kebabs with salad

Grilled tuna with grilled peppers and a green salad

Chicken Caesar salad

Suzi's Salad (see page 122)

Tomato and onion salad, small pieces of feta cheese and olives

If you need more bulk, you can add 1–2 tablespoons of the OK grains to either lunch or supper, but not both.

Snacks

A small handful of berries or one piece of fruit from the OK and good lists

A handful of sunflower and pumpkin seeds – you can have these *with* one piece of fruit to keep blood sugars even

A small handful of mixed, unsalted nuts – not *with* seeds or fruit

One oatcake or rye crispbread with cottage cheese or quark

Half an avocado with lemon juice or the recommended dressing

A boiled egg

A small piece of cheese from your daily allowance

A piece of chicken

A vegetable juice – choose one from the Detox Plan

A small smoothie, choose from chapter 13 or 15

If you are eating out a lot, use this pyramid as a guide to which proteins are the healthiest. The ones at the top are the best, the ones at the bottom the worst.

Oily fish – mackerel, salmon, herring, sardine, tuna
All other fish – shellfish and white fish
Poultry – chicken, turkey, pheasant, partridge etc
Eggs – organic and free-range
Game – choose organic and 'wild' meats such as venison, bison etc as they will be leaner
Lamb – organic wherever possible
Beef – organic wherever possible
Pork – organic wherever possible
Offal
Meat products – sausages, bacon etc

It's nearly impossible to recommend a pudding that doesn't contain lots of sugar or fruit. But if you are eating out or entertaining, here are a few suggestions:

Puddings

Strawberries and raspberries with a tablespoon of yoghurt, quark or cream
Goat's cheese and celery
Stewed apple
2 oatmeal or rye biscuits with a little cheese
A peach or a nectarine

Drinks

2 litres of water a day – minimum
One cup of black coffee, organic *or* one cup of black tea, organic
Herbal teas
Ginger and lemon in hot water
Least sugary alcohol: vodka and tequila!

Top tips in the real world

- There is no need to count calories or measure foods from the good carbs list
- Oily fish such as salmon and tuna, tinned or fresh, can be eaten as much as you like, because of the Omega 3 content.
- Eggs, whether boiled, poached or scrambled, make an excellent breakfast as they give a slow release of energy throughout the day.
- Any small amount of protein is important for the first meal of the day as it helps support the adrenals, and your energy levels, better than carbohydrates.
- Always have breakfast. Studies have shown that people who eat a nutritious breakfast, with protein and slow-releasing carbohydrate, are less likely to be hungry or overeat during the rest of the day.
- Try not to have any carbs after 6 p.m., apart from vegetables and/or your daily fruit allowance.
- Eat before 8 p.m. as the body's digestive enzymes are greatly reduced after 6 p.m.
- Don't eat nuts *with* seeds.
- But *do* eat seeds with fruit, it slows down the sugar rush.
- Take digestive enzymes with each meal and take 2 if eating supper *after* 8.00 p.m.
- IF you're still smoking, take 2–3 mg of vitamin C daily till this eating plan sorts out your blood-sugar levels.
- Don't panic if you sabotage the entire diet 2 weeks into it. It's very common to suddenly want to binge on the very things you've lived happily without – I've done it myself. Just start again the next day and don't beat yourself up about it!

You should feel and see the benefits of this eating plan within three or four weeks. Apart from losing weight, you may find that for the first time in your life you have superbly balanced blood sugars, increased energy and those chocolate cravings will be a thing of the past. Promise! Just give it a try for a minimum of a month and watch those pounds and cravings just disappear. But PLEASE avoid the foods on the 'bad carbs' list as much as you can for a minimum of *two weeks*, to get your body used to doing without its addiction.

There is one final reminder. As you may have read earlier, successful weight loss relies on synergy – 'the working together of two or more components to be more successful or productive as a result of a merger'. In other words, you need more than two components in order to lose weight successfully.

You now know what not to eat to keep the weight off, but please don't forget the other two components: exercise and the emotional level – the link between the mind and the body.

If you have all three components in place, you cannot fail to reach your optimum weight. Here's a final reminder of what you need to continue to do to get all three components working together.

CONTINUE AS MUCH AS POSSIBLE

Tibetan 5 rites – these are muscle toning and energizing exercises, so try and continue them each day. It will only take you 5 minutes and will set you up for the day.

Skin-brushing – every day before your shower. This will clear away any toxicity and dead cells that have gathered on your skin overnight.

Two litres of water a day – you can't lose weight without nature's diuretic and it will fill you up.

Four hours of exercise a week – essential if you really want to burn fat. It doesn't matter what you do, as long as you do it!

Your favourite affirmation or technique from the weekend – choose an exercise you particularly liked during the Kickstart Detox and practise it daily.

You'll find even more advice on how to live in the real world and continue with your new regime in the next chapter.

17.

Living in the Real World

Whichever plan you decided to follow, hopefully, by now, you've solved your blood-sugar highs and lows, detoxed, you feel on top of the world AND you've lost weight.

So how do you continue reaping the benefits of your new regime whilst living in the real world with all those temptations around you? To help you, here's a quick synopsis of each chapter followed by a top tip that will help you carry on eating out, entertaining and generally having a great time without the weight piling back on.

And if you do spot any old cravings coming back to haunt you, just get straight back to a day or two of detoxing as well as drinking more water. Sabotaging a detox or diet is human nature. You've followed one of the plans for a couple of weeks, feel and look wonderful and then suddenly, out of the blue, you start desperately 'needing' chocolate, coffee or a glass of wine.

It's almost as if the liver's saying, 'Hey, I'm nice and clean now, throw some toxins at me, I'm bored!' If it happens to you (and it does to me), just go with the flow, don't beat yourself up but don't let those cravings get hold of you either. Have a couple of days of 'bad' behaviour but make a determined effort to follow one of the following suggestions to get you back on track. You're only human! Remember, if you can stick to one of the plans for 80 per cent of the time and enjoy your life to the full for the other 20 per cent, you've got the perfect balance for you and your scales!

CHAPTER 3
W – weight – how to keep it off

Don't overeat

Look round a table and watch how much people eat and how quickly. I carried out this exercise for myself some time ago and noticed, for the first time in my life, that the amount of food eaten directly correlated to the size of each person. There was one overweight woman, who picked and grazed anything and everything put on the table. There was me, slimmish but carrying a few unwanted pounds. I ate everything on my plate, quickly, but stopped after finishing my meal. There was a very slim young woman who ate most but not all of her food, very, very slowly, and left what she couldn't finish. And there was a very skinny girl who hardly touched her food at all, but I'm not even going there!

> **❗ TOP TIP**
>
> Stop eating before you are full to bloating. Your stomach needs a few minutes to send signals to the brain that you're full. Give it a full 5 minutes and you won't want to eat any more.

Improve your digestion

Make sure your digestion is working as proficiently as possible by giving it a bit of help. Very often, a distended belly has more to do with how you've digested your food than with the number of calories you've consumed. You need to warn your stomach that food's on the way so it can prepare for it by producing digestive enzymes to break it down properly.

10 Top tips for a healthier digestion

1. Chew your food at least 20 times – acidic food, such as protein, will become more alkaline and easier to digest.
2. Make sure you are relaxed and always sit down.
3. Don't bolt your food down while you're on the run.
4. Make sure you're not gulping down enormous amounts of air with your food by chatting away and forgetting to chew!
5. Don't drink liquid *with* your meals.
6. Start each meal with a vegetable juice or salad to keep digestive enzymes high.
7. Eat regularly, but try to leave 4 hours between eating to allow your digestion to finish its work.
8. If you need to snack, make it fruit with a few seeds.
9. Try 1–2 glasses of water first, you could be dehydrated.
10. If all else fails, take a digestive enzyme with each meal.

CHAPTER 4
E – eliminate – in the real world

Yippee! You can now have anything from the original 'eliminate' list, but in small quantities and as a special treat. The rule of thumb is to have a little of what you fancy, but not *every* day.

Anything that is going to get your blood-sugar levels fluctuating should still be avoided as much as possible, otherwise carb- and stimulant-bingeing may start again and your body will start stashing any excess glycogen as FAT. But that doesn't mean a lifetime of avoiding your favourite food or drink, it just means anything is fine as long as it's in moderation.

I used to eat pasta practically every night. Now I eat it a couple of times a year. I just don't want it, need it or crave it – that's how much your body can change after following one of the plans for a few weeks or months.

If you're out at a restaurant with friends, by all means have a pudding. But make it one between two of you, or better still between four. Again, you may find that your sweet tooth has completely vanished, apart from the times when alcohol or PMS trigger those familiar cravings.

The higher up the following list your favourite 'baddie' is, the more it's likely to be converted straight to fat, or cause bloating, and the more you should make it an occasional or weekend treat only. The lower down the list it is, the more frequently you can have it. But try to leave 3–4 days between the foods that you *know* trigger bloating and weight gain so you don't form the same old patterns. (You could always make your own list of treats.) That way you won't start laying down fat again.

But for goodness' sake enjoy yourself, you deserve it!

Occasional treats in descending order of badness!

Sugar	Alcohol
Chocolates and Sweets	Dairy Products
Cakes and Pastries	Wheat and Pasta
Fried Food	Potatoes
Crisps	Salt
Soft Drinks	Coffee
Ready-Made Meals	Tea
Ice Cream	

 TOP TIP

If you do get an uncontrollable craving for something naughty, it may well be your blood-sugar levels hitting an all-time low. Instead of reaching for that chocolate bar, drink a glass of room temperature water instead and you will probably find the urge just goes away!

CHAPTER 5
I – incorporate – in the real world

Descending order of preferred foods

> Green Vegetables
> Other Vegetables
> Protein or Pulses
> Seeds, Nuts & Oils – EFAs
> Fruit
> Grains
> Other Carbohydrates

Green vegetables

Eat as many green vegetables as you like, they contain very few calories but masses of vitamins and minerals. Even frozen veg will do. They are going to be much higher in nutrients than fresh vegetables that have sat in your fridge for weeks.

Green vegetables will also keep your bowel clean and your blood-sugar levels even by providing plenty of fibre, as well as all the carbohydrate you need.

Don't forget yellow, orange and red vegetables either; they're full of betacarotene, a powerful antioxidant that the body converts to vitamin A for healthy hair, eyes and skin. Vegetables such as peppers and carrots are a little higher in natural sugars and starch, but you should still be able to eat them regularly without them affecting your weight, as long as you eat smaller portions than your greens and have them raw wherever possible.

Protein and pulses

You are well aware by now that eating an excessive amount of protein is not a good idea as it can cause all kinds of health problems. But a little protein is an essential part of your daily eating plan if your metabolism is to function properly and your weight is to stay stable. So make sure you eat plenty of the 'healthy' proteins such as Omega 3-rich oily fish and less of the proteins high in saturated fat such as bacon, sausages and processed meat. Watch your intake of red meat, and other non-organic meats as well, as they are high in arachidonic acid which encourages inflammation and fluid retention.

Use this list as a guide to which proteins are the best for your health and weight. The higher they appear, the more you can eat of them. The lower they appear the less you should eat.

It goes without saying that lovely crispy bacon, sausages and processed meat should be considered as very occasional treats if you want them to stay off your thighs!

> **Oily fish** – mackerel, salmon, herring, sardine, tuna
> **All other fish** – shellfish and white fish
> **Poultry** – chicken, turkey, pheasant, partridge etc
> **Eggs** – organic and free-range
> **Game** – choose organic and 'wild' meats such as venison,
>   bison etc as they will be leaner
> **Lamb** – organic wherever possible
> **Beef** – organic wherever possible
> **Pork** – organic wherever possible
> **Offal**
> **Meat products** – sausages, bacon etc

Pulses, nuts & seeds

Pulses are a very cheap source of protein, low in fat and high in fibre. They are ideal for vegetarians and vegans but need to be mixed with grains (e.g. beans on toast) in order to make them a 'complete' protein containing all eight of the essential amino acids found in animal proteins. Don't eat large amounts of pulses if you are eating fish, meat and eggs etc.

Nuts and seeds are also rich sources of protein, as well as of essential fatty acids, so can be eaten regularly. A small handful of unsalted seeds and nuts each day is a much 'slimmer' and energy-giving alternative to a chocolate bar but don't eat huge amounts unless you're not eating any animal products.

You can also sprinkle pumpkin, sesame or sunflower seeds on your yoghurt, salad or fruit salad for an extra boost of EFAs and protein.

Essential fatty acids

> Oily fish
> Seeds & nuts
> Flaxseed, hempseed, or a blended Omega 3 & 6 oil

Make sure you get plenty of 'healthy' fats every day. Essential fatty acids are so essential for every gland and organ in your body that you CAN'T lose weight without them. If you're not into oily fish, seeds and nuts, you can always kickstart your day with the smoothie suggested during the Detox Weekend in chapter 13. This will provide you with your full quota of the fat-busting Omega 3 & 6 essential fatty acids.

Fruit

Fruit is low in calories and high in antioxidants and fibre as well as being made up of 70–90 per cent water, so this is a great food for flushing fluid retention out of your system. But fruit does contain high sugar levels, albeit natural sugars, so make sure you don't overeat fruit if you want to continue to lose weight. Eat less of the starchy fruits such as bananas, and more of the watery low-sugar fruits, such as raspberries and strawberries.

 TOP TIP

Pound for pound, strawberries provide you with more vitamin C and less sugar than oranges. 100 g of strawberries, about ten, is just 27 calories. Have a handful a day instead of your usual sugar fixes.

Grains & carbs

You will probably need more grains and carbohydrate in the winter to fill you up. But for keeping the weight off, just make sure the starch content of your meal is the *smallest* part of it as you're getting enough carbs from your plentiful veg. If you are training for a marathon or a similar challenge, or work out for more than two hours a day, you will need more carbohydrate and should talk to your trainer about the amount your regime requires.

Here is a list of grains that are good alternatives to white bread and pasta. You can even find breads made from spelt or rye in most shops nowadays. If wheat isn't causing you a problem you can have wholegrain bread and pasta instead, but bear in mind that if you're not burning your carbs off you'll end up wearing them so keep the portions small in relation to vegetables and protein.

> **Brown Rice**
> **Quinoa**
> **Millet**
> **Spelt**
> **Rye**
> **Wholewheat Bread & Pasta**

❗ TOP TIP

If you eat a sandwich or a bowl of pasta for lunch, your body needs to hold on to the equivalent of 3 cups of water to be able to convert the starch to glycogen to be stored. Result? An expanding waistline and a huge energy slump. If you know you're going to have a starchy meal, make sure you drink 1 pint of water an hour beforehand to help it on its way.

Water

Finally, don't forget to drink at least 2 litres of water a day. Water helps you lose weight by eliminating fluid retention, and filling you up. You can't lose weight without it. It will also flush toxins out, give you more energy, lovely skin and make sure you 'eliminate' regularly. Try and drink STILL natural mineral water at room temperature. You'll drink more if it's not fizzy. Drink a glass of water for every cup of coffee or glass of wine you drink. Make it two. And keep a bottle on your desk to make sure you're getting through your 2 litres a day.

! TOP TIP

Set an hourly alarm on your computer or watch and, every hour on the hour, drink a standard-sized glass of water. That way you will easily get through 8–10 glasses a day.

CHAPTER 6
G – get up and go – exercising in the real world

When it comes to keeping the weight off, getting enough exercise is as important as your eating regime.

If you do nothing else, start each day with the 5 Rites you learned during the Kickstart Detox weekend. And, when you can, try and fit in an exercise class, yoga or a brisk walk. For continued weight loss this should be 4–5 times a week. If that's impossible, make sure to build at least 20 minutes of glow-inducing exercise into each day. And if you can't do that, at least get up and move around as much as possible during a sedentary day.

People who walk instead of drive, go up stairs instead of taking the lift, and run around after toddlers all day, are usually slimmer and fitter than gym bunnies who sweat it out three times a week but spend the rest of the time being couch potatoes!

10 Top tips for building more exercise into your day

1. Walk up the stairs instead of taking the lift.
2. Walk up escalators.
3. Park the car at the furthest end of the car park.
4. Get off the bus a couple of stops early.
5. Walk to post a letter, buy a newspaper etc.
6. Walk fast enough to break out in a slight sweat.
7. Use a basket for shopping instead of a trolley.
8. Put the radio on and have a dance while waiting for the kettle to boil.
9. Stand up on the train, bus or Tube instead of sitting.
10. Hide TV remote control so you have to get up to change channels.

CHAPTER 7
H – holistic therapies – do one regularly

There are so many therapies you can try out to help you fight the flab, expel the toxins and keep your lymph moving. But if you do just one, I would recommend a colonic irrigation from time to time. It will help your large intestine prevent bad bacteria from breeding and gets rid of months of toxicity. I have never met anyone who doesn't rave about clearer skin, weight loss and a nice flat tummy following one. More importantly, it will improve your bowel action so food doesn't start backing up again and cause bloating. So be brave, and try a colonic, if you haven't already. Colonics are particularly useful after Christmas, when the seasons change, or before a special event. Try and follow a mini-detox for a week before booking one.

If you don't fancy the idea of a colonic, have a look at chapter 7 on holistic therapies, and make sure you get a regular massage or treatment at your local beauty salon. Anything that gets the lymph moving will help you keep the weight off. If you have the time, but don't have the money, there is bound to be a local college needing 'guinea pigs' for its courses. Check out what's on offer and put yourself on the list. You will be charged very little in return for being practised on.

▌TOP TIP

The most important thing you can do for your body to help get the toxicity out is to keep your lymph moving, so make sure you skin-brush every day. It only takes 5 minutes before you jump in the shower each morning. See chapter 13 on how to skin-brush.

CHAPTER 8
T – toxins – how to cope in the real world

You're in the real world now, so you can't go about your normal day hiding from your mobile phone, Tube travel and a stressful job.

What you can do is to make sure you keep the internal and external toxins to an absolute minimum and get enough rest and relaxation to combat all the stresses of life.

5 Top tips

1. **Reduce toxins that over-stimulate the adrenals: salt, sugar, cigarettes, tea, coffee, and alcohol.** In excess they produce too much blood glucose which, if not used up, is quickly turned to fat.
2. **Try to avoid stress as much as possible.** Apart from over-stimulating the adrenals, prolonged stress also causes food intolerances, digestive disorders and a toxic build-up, which can account for pounds of excess weight in the form of undigested food and water retention.
3. **Get enough sleep.** You're more likely to get carb cravings if you're tired, so try and get enough sleep. If you are

asleep by 11 p.m. the rest you get during this hour is three times deeper than you get *after* midnight.

4. **Eat natural food whenever possible.** Your entire diet doesn't have to be organic, but remember that fat cells LOVE toxins, so keep the chemicals found in non-organic food, ready-made meals and over-the-counter drugs to a minimum.

5. **Allow yourself a little 'me' time each day.** Give yourself 10 minutes off for: meditation, relaxation, yoga, T'ai Chi, or just a walk in nature. The less stress and toxicity in your system, the less fat is accumulated.

CHAPTER 9
L – liver – how to support it in the real world

Your liver is involved in carb-, fat- and protein metabolism, so you want it working as well as it can to keep your metabolism on an even keel. It can't do its job properly if stimulants, toxins and stress constantly bombard it.

So anything that is considered by the liver to be an enemy, whether it's too much caffeine, nicotine, alcohol or sugar, or too many pesticides, additives and chemicals, needs to be eliminated as much as possible if your liver's going to help you keep slim.

! TOP TIP – DAILY LIVER FLUSH JUICE

Beetroot, radishes and watercress, in particular, help drain your liver by stimulating your gall bladder. Juice one small beetroot, 4 radishes and a small bunch of watercress. Add a quarter of a lemon, with a little of the pith, a small chunk of ginger and a couple of carrots. Drink immediately.

If you haven't a juicer or don't have enough time, add half a freshly squeezed lemon and a little grated ginger to a glass or two of warm water and drink on an empty stomach. This will kickstart your digestion and liver.

CHAPTER 10

O – oedema – water retention – how to avoid it in the real world

Many things can cause water retention, from hormones in birth control pills to HRT, too much salt or too many stimulants. Here's a brief reminder of the things that can cause water retention and how to avoid it in the real world.

Dehydration – the body will hold on to excess water if you don't drink enough. Make sure you drink 2 litres of water a day.

Constipation – if your colon isn't getting rid of waste at least once a day (preferably twice) your body is more likely to retain fluid to dilute the partially digested foods still stuck in your gut. Add the recommended colon cleanser to your daily regime if things aren't moving enough.

EFA deficiency – too few EFAs and the body is more likely to retain excess fluid. Eat oily fish, seeds and nuts or take one tablespoon of the recommended Omega 3 & 6 oils daily.

Sugar & carbohydrate excess – balancing your blood-sugar levels will prevent excess weight being stored as water. Keep sugar and refined carbohydrates to a minimum – which includes alcohol.

Sodium excess – too much salt forces the body to hold on to extra amounts of water to dilute the sodium and the tissues become waterlogged. Check the labelling of every single product you buy for sodium content.

Stimulants – every cup of tea, coffee, soft drink or alcoholic drink encourages your body to mobilize about three cups of water to remove the stimulants.

Toxins – the body retains water to keep toxic material away from your vital organs – which is why you can look so puffy. Avoid toxins as much as you can.

> ❗ **TOP TIP**
>
> Dried dandelion leaf tea is one of the best ways to help the kidneys remove water from your body. For temporary water retention, such as just before a period or a special event, you can drink two to four cups of dandelion leaf tea a day.

CHAPTER 11
S – synergy – tap your subconscious

Spend a couple of minutes a day repeating one of your favourite affirmations. I still look in the mirror on a daily basis and say, 'Gosh, my thighs are getting slimmer', instead of homing in on the negative! Keep doing it: the power we have over our unconscious is quite remarkable.

> ❗ **TOP TIP**
>
> Try saying these words over and over again just for a couple of days. Allow them to fill your consciousness. Repeat them for several days. Don't worry about 'how' to accomplish it or 'when' it will happen. Trust the intelligence within you and believe that you *deserve* whatever it is you wish for – including weight loss!
>
> **Everything I touch is a success, including weight loss.**

CHAPTER 12

S – supplements – which one to take in the real world

Any of the supplements you have tried and enjoyed or, for a good all-rounder, I would recommend Detoxil to anyone living in the real world, leading a stressful life, drinking or smoking or living in a city. In fact, just living! It will help support your liver in its daily battle with toxins as well as protecting your immunity.

Detoxil consists of 26 bio-active nutrients, including: carotenoids, amino acids, vitamins C, E and vitamin B-complex plus natural diuretics dandelion and artichoke that work together to eliminate toxicity.

It also contains zinc for insulin metabolism, copper, iron, phosphatidylcholine for helping the liver break down fat, and grapefruit extract, which is an anti-fungal agent for a healthy bowel. It's a good all-round multivitamin and liver protector.

Details of where to buy it can be found under Resources at the back of the book.

As I said at the beginning of the book, losing weight and keeping that weight off is not rocket science: eat less and exercise more. I hope you have now discovered for yourself that there are a lot of other little things we can do each day that will help prevent fluid retention, toxicity, stress AND weight gain.

If you treat the suggestions in this book as essential weapons in your battle against unwanted fat, you'll win the war! Permanently. But never forget life is for living, so:

80 per cent weight-loss programme + 20 per cent a little of what you fancy = optimum weight

20 Top tips for living in the real world

1. Chew, chew chew. Chewing tells the digestion to start producing enzymes so your food is better digested. And better digestion equals less weight.

2. Keep enzymes high by starting each meal with a raw salad.

3. Eat your largest meal of the day as close to midday as possible. You are more likely to burn it off.

4. Always have breakfast to keep your metabolism ticking over.

5. Eat your lightest meal in the evening, preferably before 8 p.m.

6. Enforce a 6 p.m. curfew on starches and carbohydrates.

7. Use smaller plates so you eat smaller portions.

8. Only eat when you are truly hungry.

9. Go food shopping *after* you've eaten.

10. If you fall off the wagon, get right back on and don't beat yourself up.

11. Only weigh yourself every couple of weeks.

12. Allow an indulgence a couple of times a week and enjoy it!

13. Only eat what you can hold in two hands. Two cupped hands equal three quarters of your stomach size.

14. Do a 'liquid only' day once a week to help your body keep losing weight. Have a smoothie, soup and juice day.

15. Have a no-protein day twice a week, having just vegetables and salads on those days.

16. A meal doesn't have to be a banquet. You don't need a starter, main course and pudding all at one meal. Don't send the stomach too many messages at one go, it can't cope!

17. SWEAT every day, to get the toxins out: garden, exercise, make love, whatever it takes for a minimum of 20 minutes a day!

18. Do yoga or T'ai Chi exercises in the evening.

19. Find 5–20 minutes a day to relax the body and mind.

20. Do a positive affirmation every day. It works!

Appendix

The Barnes axial temperature test

The most accurate measurement of thyroid activity is the body's basal (resting) temperature, which reflects your metabolic rate – the rate at which the body converts food into energy for fuel. Your thyroid sets the metabolic rate, so if your thyroid function is low, so is your basal temperature.

All you need is a mercury thermometer to measure your armpit temperature. Before you go to sleep, shake the thermometer and leave it by the bed. On waking, before doing anything else, place it in your armpit and wait a full 10 minutes. Record the temperature. Repeat for at least 5 days to obtain an average.

Men and post-menopausal women can take their temperature on any day, as long as they are not running a temperature.

Women who are still experiencing menstruation will have fluctuating temperatures because of their hormonal cycles, so it is advisable to do this test on the second, third, and fourth day of your period.

Normal body temperature in the morning is between 36.6 and 36.8°C (97.8 to 98.2°F). A temperature that is 36.4°C or LESS (97.4°F) suggests that you may have low thyroid function.

Solution

As well as the recommended eating plans and supplements, the most important mineral is iodine, an essential component of the thyroid hormones which you can take safely in the form of kelp or dulse. Kelp is very gentle in its effect on the thyroid and it also helps bind to toxins such as heavy metals and carry them out of the body, so is a useful tool for detoxing. But if you are already under medication for a poor thyroid then please *don't* take kelp or dulse without discussing with your doctor first. And if you are at all worried, please see your doctor. Here are some other suggestions:

- Reduce coffee, black tea and alcohol.
- Drink plenty of water.
- Eat plenty of deep-sea fish, such as shellfish, cod, bass and haddock, for its rich iodine content.
- Sprinkle iodine-rich Nori flakes, seaweed, and dulse or kelp on to your food.
- Increase your Essential Fatty Acid consumption.
- Don't overeat: peanuts, Brussels sprouts, broccoli, kale, cauliflower or soya products. They can affect iodine absorption.
- And follow one of the three plans, incorporating all of the above!

Acknowledgements

A big thank you to all the experts who provided me with a wealth of information and quotes and, in particular, to Udo Erasmus, Stuart Tranter, Vanessa Ough, Penny May, Nor Power and Dr Shamim Daya for their valuable contributions; to Kate Adams, Sarah Day, Elisabeth Merriman, Myra Jones, Georgina Atsiaris, Clare Pollock, and everyone at Penguin for their support, enthusiasm and editorial improvements; to my agent Ruth for her non-stop encouragement; to my brother David and my friends and family, in London and Brighton, for their undying faith in me. Finally, thank you to all my clients for having inspired me in the first place. Keep up the good work!

Resources

Further Reading

Udo Erasmus, *Fats that Heal, Fats that Kill* (Alive Books)

Udo Erasmus, *Choosing the Right Fats* (Alive Books)

Dr Johanna Budwig, *Flax Oil as a True Aid Against Arthritis, Heart Infarction, Cancer and Other Diseases* (Apple Publishing)

T. K. V. Desikachar, *The Heart of Yoga: Developing a Personal Practice* (Inner Traditions International)

Kiew Kit Wong, *The Complete Book of Tai Chi Chuan: A Comprehensive Guide to the Principles and Practice* (Vermilion)

Louise L. Hay, *You Can Heal Your Life* (Eden Grove Editions)

Joseph Goldstein, Sharon Salzberg, *Insight Meditation Kit: A Step-by-step Course on How to Meditate* (Sounds True Audio)

Organizations and Experts

Suzi Grant: www.benatural.co.uk

British Association for Nutritional Therapy: www.bant.org.uk

BMI index: www.bbc.co.uk/health/yourweight/bmi.shtml

Allergy UK: www.allergyuk.org tel: 020 8303 8525

Plaskett Nutritional Medicine College: www.pnmcollege.com

Professor Loren Cordain, PhD, Department of Health and Exercise Science, Colorado State University: www.thepaleodiet.com

The Food Commission: www.foodcomm.org.uk

Yoga Haven: www.yogahaven.co.uk

Vanessa Ough, aromatherapist: positivehealth@btopenworld.com

Wayne Leonard, Hogarth Health Club: www.thehogarth.co.uk tel: 020 8995 4600

Penny May, T'ai Chi instructor: penny@madasafish.com
General T'ai Chi website: www.another-voice.net

Suppliers

Organic essential oils are available from 'Materia Aromatica'. An unscented 'Body Milk' is also exclusive to them: www.materia-aromatica.com tel: 020 8392 9868

For Udo's Choice oil blend, Beyond Greens and Digestive Enzymes: Savant Distribution, www.savant-health.com tel: 08450 60 60 70

For milk thistle, kelp and tasteless flaxseed oil etc: Nutrigold, www.nutrigold.co.uk tel: 01884 251777

For Valdivia natural sugar and Nature et Progrès Seasalt: The Wholistic Medical Centre, tel: 020 7580 7537

Detoxil is available from major pharmacies and health food stores at a retail price of £7.95 for 30 tablets, at the time of going to print: www.detoxil.com

Index